CW00809367

MIRROR OF THE BODY

Your Mouth Reflects the Health
of Your Whole Body

By
James E. Rota, DDS

Disclaimer Note to the Reader:

Although the author and publisher have exhaustively researched all sources to ensure the accuracy and completeness of the information contained in this book, we assume no responsibility for errors, inaccuracies, omissions or any inconsistency herein. Any slights of people, places or organizations are unintentional. The views and opinions expressed in this book are only those of the author.

You assume full responsibility and risk or loss resulting from information in this book. The publisher and author will not be liable for any special, indirect, incidental, consequential, or punitive damages or any other damages whatsoever, whether in an action of contract, statute, tort (including negligence) or otherwise, relating to the use of information herein. Certain links within the book lead to resources maintained by third parties over whom the author and publisher have no control, and the author and publisher make no representations or warranties as to the accuracy of those resources.

The information contained in this book are based on research and the personal and professional experience of the author. This book has been published for information and references only. It is not intended in any respect as a substitute for a visit to a qualified dentist, physician, or other licensed health care practitioner. If you have a dental or medical problem, please consult a qualified dentist, physician or health care provider for diagnosis and treatment under their supervision. The publisher and author are not responsible for any adverse effects or consequences resulting from the use of any suggestions, procedures, protocols, or remedies discussed in this book.

Cover Design by Dori Rota
Epilogue Contribution by Shirley Fretto
Printed by CreateSpace
Available from Amazon.com and other retail outlets

ISBN 978-0975954904

Copyright 2015 by James E. Rota, DDS

All Rights Reserved. Printed and bound in the United States of America. No part of this book may be reproduced in any form or by any means, electronic or mechanical, including photocopying, recording or otherwise without the written consent of the copyright holder.

Dedication

To Shirley, my best friend and angel, whose integrity, loyalty, and unconditional love saved me from myself throughout my life.

To my loving wife, Dori, whose devotion to our mission has been carried out with passion, perseverance, and purpose.

To my patients, for whom I have deeply cared, and felt honored to be a part of their quest for wellness.

Table of Contents

Acknowledgements

I sincerely hesitate to accept credit for the accomplishment in writing this book – especially after reviewing its contents and retracing my journey through the profession of dentistry. I am blessed to have been a part of the evolution of dentistry, as it included my own evolvement of who and what I am during my pursuit of optimum health.

I want to acknowledge the people in my life who greatly influenced my development. My grade school teacher, Sister Rose Michael, inspired me to trust my ability to learn. She taught me that I could have anything if I want it badly enough. "What the mind can conceive and believe, it will achieve." With those words indelibly scribed in the back of my mind, I pursued my dental education.

At the Loyola University School of Dentistry, I was fortunate to have Dr. Paul Dawson as an instructor. He recommended me to Dr. Robert Wolcott, a research dentist in the US Navy. This introduction to Dr. Wolcott changed the course of my life. He brought me on as an Assistant Professor at the UCLA School of Dentistry as it was forming. With the support of my first wife, Dolores, and my children, I was able to accept this position and flourish in my career.

As a dentist, finding a truly synergistic partner to carry out the important work at the dental chair while putting the patient at ease is a true blessing. I was fortunate to have two such assistants, Pam Wilson and Scott Chavez. Pam came to me in the 1970s and worked with me for 20 years. Sadly, she passed away in 2001, of breast cancer. She was an example to all dental assistants. Her confidence and ability to anticipate, made my job easier and more productive. Scott Chavez is a true champion in dentistry, patient care, and education. His compassion, wisdom and integrity brought a standard of care to our office for many years that was greatly appreciated by myself and our patients. He facilitated the development of the dental practice as a partner in the later years, and shared my passion for biological dentistry. I am exceedingly grateful.

In my evolution as a dentist, I am thankful for the dedication to truth and science by the International Academy of Oral Medicine and Toxicology. It was the integrity and intellect of people like Michael Ziff, his father Sam, David Kennedy, Joyal Taylor, and

Walter "Jess" Clifford that drew me to the path of biological dentistry and assisted me in my journey.

Pioneer dentists, such as Dr. Hal Huggins, DDS, were oppressed as they became vocal about the truth of mercury fillings. They endured the undeserved castigation in spite of speaking the truth. I also acknowledge the mercury poisoned victims who speak out for those who can't speak for themselves or do not yet know the truth. These are some of the people whom I have witnessed perseverance in the face of injustice: Leo Cashman, Freya Koss, Dawn Ewing, Kelly Gallagher, Randall Moore, Marisa Russo, Anita Tibau, Bernie Windham, Marie Flowers, Kristin Mills, Charlie Brown, Tom McGuire, Robert Cartland, and Amanda Just. To everyone doing their part in mercury awareness, I am grateful.

My final acknowledgment goes to my best friends: Shirley Fretto and Dori Rota. As my office manager and confidant for more than forty years, I have always relied on Shirley. It is fair to say that some patients were probably more excited to come to the office to see Shirley than for me. There are no words I could say or act of acknowledgment I could do that would approach the amount of gratitude and love I have for this outstanding person.

My wife, Dori, has worked with me closely throughout this entire book and contributed her flavor to the subject matter, after attending numerous lectures and conferences for the past thirteen years. She has truly loved me throughout our "adventure," and makes it easy for me to love her in return. Dori's passion, technical skills and eclectic talents have been instrumental in making my dreams come to reality.

"All truth passes through three stages:
First, it is ridiculed, second it is violently opposed,
and third it is accepted as self-evident."
Arthur Schopenhauer, 19th Century Philosopher

Introduction

In writing this book, I am reminded of the many times in my professional career I have sat down to write a book regarding some phase of my accumulating experiences in dentistry. One of the things I enjoyed most in my career was sharing new and exciting health discoveries with my patients. Because I was personally growing, along with my profession, there was always more to learn and more to share. I kept putting it off until I thought, someday, I will include all of the latest techniques and scientific revelations regarding the health of this wondrous, most sensitive place of our human anatomy, our mouth. I soon discovered that our mouth was a mirror reflecting the health or disease of our body and mind, which I found most fascinating as I examined thousands of patients. I thought one day I would share these revelations, and I am, but this is not a book simply about dentistry.

I have been practicing dentistry for fifty-plus years. It is a "practice" in the literal sense in that we are repeating and learning in order to improve our performance. We may even gain wisdom along the course of our service. We have been told by Hermes, that "When the Student is Ready, the Teacher will Appear." Well, the reverse was also stated, "When the Teacher is Ready, the Student will Appear." I trust that both of us are ready since this book has appeared and you are reading this message. I am confident that the information in this book will change your life as it did mine; not just about your mouth, but your entire body, mind, and attitude about life.

During the course of my career, I had been exposed, on a daily basis, to an abundance of physical and emotional stress and toxic materials associated with the restoration of the mouth. Due to the exposure to mercury used in silver amalgam fillings and other toxic materials, I have had my share of health challenges. "A terrible sin against humanity" (a statement made by the world-renown inorganic chemist, Dr. Alfred Stock), refers to the dental mercury amalgam filling, which has been the commonly placed filling in this country since the 1800s.

I had been unknowingly affected by mercury, including the replacement of old, broken down silver amalgam fillings. I was not aware that the removal of the old filling resulted in the creation of mercury vapor, which is absorbed by the lungs and nasal passages and is as toxic as elemental mercury. These vapors not only affected the health of our patient, but also the dental team. Dental assistants are also directly in contact with mercury and its toxic vapor. These properties of mercury can greatly undermine the nervous system and the immune system, making us more prone to illness, depending upon our own susceptibility.

Throughout this book, I will share how I met those challenges and how they served me in finding a way of life that promotes optimal physical health and has allowed me to be in better health mentally and spiritually today than in my forties. Now, at the age of 81, while I am no longer practicing chairside dentistry, I continue service to others by sharing my uncommon story.

This book is intended for everyone; anyone that has or ever had teeth. While there are a few passages in this book that may be more meaningful to a dentist, I feel it is important to communicate these ideas, which may benefit them in their own practice. Many dentists don't see beyond the drilling, filling and billing. I was fortunate enough to be part of the evolution of dentistry since the 1960s, developing commonplace dental procedures and equipment advances to discovering the holistic connection of the mouth to the rest of the body ... and spirit.

I do not intend to frighten you about the harmful effects of mercury or the other health challenges that our body experiences from day to day.

This book is about learning what you can do about it and all of the things that threaten this wonderful, forgiving body of ours. It does have the capacity to heal itself from the most challenging circumstances, once we learn its extraordinary capacity.

10

This is a book about hope, not only for you and me, but for mankind. I sincerely feel that the toxins in our bodies have a gravely detrimental effect on the state of affairs of mankind. How we feel affects how we think; how we think affects how we act; and how we act as a society affects our nation and our planet as a whole.

Dr. James E. Rota

ATTENTION SKEPTICS:

If you are currently skeptical about the dangers of amalgam fillings, I understand it may be difficult to read information contrary to what you already believe. I encourage you to first read Chapter 12, "Show Me the Science," which may assist you in understanding the premise of any "controversial" statements in other chapters. Then go back and start at the beginning of the book. This approach may make the experience more palatable for you.

Chapter 1

My Toxic Sock Drawer

The heavy trap door in the floor was the least of my worries as we descended down the creaky wooden stairs into the darkness. Two dim light beams coming from small windows near the ceiling, faintly illuminated the gloomy, damp basement of my cousin's house. In the shadows, Conrad turned and said, "You gotta see this." I didn't know what treasure could be worth enduring the frightening surroundings of this forgotten and probably forbidden room.

It was 1946. My older cousin Conrad had always been a bit of a troublemaker. But that was part of the attraction. Besides, I was thrilled that a boy his age would even hang out with a twelve year old, and let me call him "Conny."

This basement was the kind most Midwestern children remember for its mystery of the unknown – unfamiliar odors, horror movie lighting, cobwebs, and the big black monster with all its tentacles, also known as the furnace.

On this fateful day, Conny reached to a top shelf of a dirty old cabinet, bringing down a bottle, to share its mysterious contents with me. Placing it in my hand, it was the most curious thing I had ever seen. I held the bottle. It was small but heavy and seemed alive. I moved my hand from side to side and watched a thick, silvery liquid inside. It was strange that such a small amount of liquid could weigh more than a pound.

Conny removed the tightly closed cap and said, "Here, stick your finger in it." I hesitated for a moment, but my cousin was four years older and seemingly wiser. So after a short period of observation, I slowly immersed my finger into the strange substance. I expected the material to feel wet, but it felt different from any liquid I had experienced. When I took my finger out, it was completely dry and without evidence of any material on my hand. "Wow, what is that?" I said, forgetting about the fearsome setting of the basement.

"It's mercury. Do you want it?" Conny whispered.
I responded enthusiastically, "Sure, I'll take it!"

Today, if we had spilled that mercury, by law, the National Response Center would be contacted, and a Hazardous Materials team would be immediately deployed.

I did not know what I was going to do with the bottle of mercury, but I had an inquisitive mind, and I looked forward to experimenting with it. At the time, I had no idea of the lethal nature of this strange substance and the consequences of my curiosity. I also did not have any idea that this substance would become an integral part of my life. This was my first introduction to a material that is known to be one of the most toxic metals on the face of this planet.

I took my liquid treasure home and placed it in the top drawer of my bureau, which was a sock drawer. Each day, while retrieving a fresh pair of stockings, I would notice the vial of liquid. The top was loosely fitted on the small container. Some of the liquid had come out of the vial, and I would watch the silvery drops move at the bottom of my drawer. From time to time, I would play with this deceptively friendly liquid metal on the floor or on the table. I found it very intriguing to see how the separated drops would come together in a most mesmerizing way to form one large mass.

I found rubbing the mercury on a penny fascinating, as it soon appeared silver. The mercury would cling and amalgamate to the copper penny. In time, I watched the oxidation process turn the penny darker in color.

For a Confirmation gift, I received a gold watch. I placed the gold watch in my sock drawer. One day I noticed the gold on the watch had been stained and corroded, and the watch stopped working. I had no idea that the mercury was responsible. It had amalgamated to the gold, creating a disfigured watch, which I eventually discarded. I did not know at the time, that the lethal colorless, odorless vapor from the mercury would greatly affect my health.

I soon began suffering from many allergies. I would often sneeze and have trouble sleeping or strange dreams. I had difficulty awakening and felt fatigued in the morning, often complaining of stomach upset and constipation. I missed many days of school. The doctors had diagnosed my allergies as hay fever, and I had to endure a series of injections which did not seem to remedy my sneezing, constipation, and watery eyes. No one had suspected or suggested that mercury could have been responsible for my early allergies and morning fatigue conditions.

When I was in the classroom, I was lethargic, had a short attention span, and difficulty remembering instructions. My symptoms today would have been commonly diagnosed as Attention Deficit Disorder (ADD).

Fortunately, I developed a close relationship with an understanding teaching nun while attending St. Patrick's Grade School in Joliet, Illinois. Years later, Sister Rose Michael shared with me that she had seen some potential in me in spite of my illness. She encouraged and supported me during those trying times. The effects of my "mercury playmate" had begun to interfere with my cognitive skills and memory retention.

Because of my learning difficulties, I decided that college would be too challenging. I enjoyed working with my hands and became interested in the industrial arts and shop courses. I had no intention of taking college preparatory courses. However, when I received an award given by the Industrial Arts Department, my advisors encouraged me to take some Junior College courses and consider enrolling in Engineering College.

I started my college education as an engineering student in Fort Wayne, at the Indiana Institute of Technology studying mechanical engineering. However, I was a long way from home and Dolores, my high school sweetheart – and combined with a lack of enthusiasm for engineering, I dropped out and headed back home after one semester.

Dolores' employer, the town dentist, also influenced my decision to leave engineering school. He suggested that I consider putting the skills of my hands and mind to good work as a dentist. I did not relish the idea of putting my hands in people's mouths. However, he said that I would learn to deal with some of my reservations, and that I would soon enjoy this profession. To be frank, the fact that Dr. Drenning and his wife lived in the affluent part of town and drove a Cadillac was also part of the intrigue.

Armed with this new motivation, I enrolled at the local junior college, and began my course of education to earn a degree in chemistry. I moved out of my parents' home, married Dolores, and made my way into adulthood, full of hope and ambition.

The contents of my toxic sock drawer stayed intact from the age of twelve until I got married, leaving my boyhood and toxic friend behind. By the time I was in college, I was married and living in a different residence. I was no longer under the chronic exposure of the mercury rolling around in my bureau drawer. I began to excel in my studies, and many of the acute symptoms began to subside.

My undergraduate work turned out to be an exceptional experience for me. I learned essential study habits, making school an easier process for me. In addition to biological and zoological course requirements, I took a lot of chemistry courses and loved it. General chemistry, inorganic chemistry, organic chemistry, qualitative analysis, quantitative analysis – the instructors were great, and I was tempted to go into chemistry as a profession. However, while getting my education, I was also building my family. I was married with two children and another on the way. I was anxious to get my degree and apply to dental school so I could provide for my growing family.

When I received my DDS degree in 1961 from the Loyola University School of Dentistry in Chicago, I had no idea that my profession would not only allow me to serve and excel in the art and science of dentistry, but it would also permit me to see myself from a larger perspective, to work with my body and with my mind – and, yes, to help me to become a better person by finding that I was part of a greater, more spiritual self.

Chapter 2

Navy Dentist Who Never Set Foot on a Ship

In 1957, I was accepted to the Loyola University School of Dentistry in Chicago. Being accepted to Dental School was a tremendous accomplishment for me. My parents were far from wealthy, so I worked my way through school. In the summer months, I worked on construction jobs. During the school year, I worked as a salesman in the electrical department at Sears Roebuck. I also had a job at a blood bank, drawing blood. At that time, I was married and had four children. (We were trying to be good Catholics.) I was determined to finish school and graduated in 1961. I was fortunate to receive the highest honor – The C.N. Johnson Award, which is only occasionally awarded since it is conferred upon a student considered to have exceptional clinical and surgical skills.

Upon graduating from dental school, I was ready to start private practice and provide for my large family of six. I was also offered a teaching position. However, our country was drafting its young citizens into the armed forces. I had a college deferment and assumed that having four children would pardon my requirement entirely. My draft board gave me the option of selecting either the Air Force or Navy and said that I would be required to honor my obligations. I selected the Navy Dental Corps. I was commissioned as a First Lieutenant and assigned to Great Lakes Naval Training Center, a recruit basic training center located in Illinois. So we packed up our meager belongings and headed to Great Lakes, Illinois, where I served in the Navy for two years. This choice later proved to be a very pivotal and fortuitous decision for me.

The Navy Dental Corps offered an internship program that allowed us to train in revolving specialty departments. This was an opportunity that I gladly received as part of my education. My salary as a First Lieutenant was also a welcomed addition to our family. We rented a small house in Mundelein, Illinois, a small town near the base, and I drove home every day with the exception of weekly duty nights.

Although I welcomed the training in each specialty of dentistry, the surgical extraction specialty was very unappealing to me. This specialty included extracting hundreds of teeth from young teenage boys, whose diet consisted of morning colas and some sweet rolls. The experience is still a dark, disheartening picture in my mind – especially one particular memory.

I remember receiving a phone call around 3 a.m. while on night duty. I had a painful wrist from extracting nearly 100 teeth that day. The call was from a technician on duty at the surgical barracks who needed help with a recruit whose hemorrhage from the afternoon extractions had not stopped.

After a driver took me to the barracks, I entered the building and the technician greeted me and escorted me down the center isle of two long rows of bunks occupied with recruits who had undergone multiple extractions that day and required hospitalization. It was a hot morning, and I was wearing the traditional officer uniform that the recruits were trained to respond with the prompt respect. The duty dental technician informed me that a young recruit had all of his teeth pulled earlier that day. The tech had attempted to change his pressure bandage a number of times but the hemorrhage persisted. The recruit's mouth was filled with a large, bloody gauze pack. There were stains on the sheet and pillowcase, and the recruit was letting out muffled sobs. It broke my heart. Since I was not only a dentist but an officer, he attempted to salute. But the technician said sternly, "Not necessary, recruit."

It was a warm summer night, and the room had no air conditioning. We were near the lake, and the humidity was high. I recall a nauseating odor permeated the area. After washing my hands in the nearby sink, I went over to remove the bloody gauze. The odor was putrefying, and it was all I could do to keep my composure and officer facade. I could see that all of his teeth had been removed and a suture had been placed to close the areas left by the extractions.

After I carefully replaced the pressure bandage, I sat down by his bed and placed my hands over his. I began to reassure him that everything would turn out fine and his rotting teeth, which had troubled him for many years, would no longer bother him. He appeared to respond, and I could see him beginning to relax. We spoke for a short time and I replaced the gauze again noting that the blood was beginning to coagulate. I assured him with a momentary squeeze of his shoulder that the healing was progressing as expected but I would be on call if he needed me. He appeared to show gratitude, but the image of him broke my heart.

I went back to my barracks and tried to sleep but couldn't get the image or the odor out of my mind. To this day, I am troubled by this recollection.

I would like to think those scenes are not taking place today. However, after examining hundreds of mouths of young recruits from all over the country and inquiring about their lifestyle, I realized there is a large number of young people whose teeth are rampantly decaying as a result of diets consisting primarily of processed carbohydrates and sugars. The attraction is not only sweets but that junk food is fast and cheap. Many had money issues, so they chose the cheaper more addictive foods. However, in the long run, who knows how costly that choice would be?

Back then, however, I wasn't as philosophical about the condition of the mouths of those in service to this country, as I was thankful to have the experience of practicing my new profession. My services were appreciated and required a lot of my attention. I also was able to provide for my family.

But I was troubled. I was considered good with my hands and my peers had acknowledged me for the quality of my restorative service, but would my expectations for the quality of my services interfere with the practical requirements of providing for a growing family? Could I develop the necessary proficiency to produce more with the same quality when I went into private practice?

I began to review literature and studies to determine if there were other dentists who shared my concern and what they were doing about it. We had no instruction regarding efficiencies and business practices of the profession in dental school. This matter required extra examination and study. At the time, there were dentists who shared my concern. I recall reading time-motion studies done by Harold Kilpatrick, who eventually wrote a book entitled, "Work Simplification in Dental Practice: Applied Time and Motion Studies in Dentistry."

While in the Navy Dental Corps, we were assigned technicians to assist us in our services. They were mostly trained to seat and release the patients, clean up afterwards and supply the necessary instruments that the dentist required. Some assistants would stand as close to the dentist as possible and attempt to be of service; however, the instrument delivery system was an obstacle for this exchange. There was a large tray near or over the patient that was used to exchange these instruments.

After reviewing the various time-motion studies conducted by doctors like Dr. Kilpatrick, I reviewed with my technician assistant some of the efficiencies of movement and design that could be incorporated into our restorative procedures. We had no choice but to deal with the equipment and develop a proficient exchange system around some of the equipment obstacles. Nevertheless, we were still able to maintain our quality of service and to increase our productivity.

We soon discovered that our efficiency work was quite timely with the Commanding Officer's orders to increase our restorative productivity to satisfy the needs of the submarine recruiting program. At the time, our government was at odds with the Russians. It was right before the Cuban Missile Crisis, and the United States was preparing for war. Our dental unit from Great Lakes was on the Florida shore during the infamous exchange between President John F. Kennedy and Russian President Nikita Khrushchev. I recall being in a church near the Florida base, praying as we listened for missiles to fly overhead.

The crisis encouraged the preparation of the submarine recruits for training with restored teeth. Our Commanding Officer required us to increase our productivity by using a temporary filling called a cement alloy. This was a mixture of 50% zinc oxy-phosphate cement with 50% of the alloy used to make the common amalgam filling, but without the mercury. In other words, the Navy was testing a mercury-free filling!

The Navy Commanders believed this would reduce considerable time in the restorative service but only provide the recruit with a "temporary" restoration. Some dentists, including myself, believed we would be doing a disservice by placing inferior fillings, which was not in keeping with our education. By using the Kilpatrick proficiency methods with our services, we felt we would satisfy the restorative production requirements using the mercury amalgam filling, resulting in a better, more permanent filling.

Therefore, a study began involving the placement of a cement alloy versus the common mercury-silver alloy.

I find it hard to justify now, but my conviction at the time was that I would be doing a disservice by placing the "inferior" cement alloy. Little did I know that I was doing a greater disservice by placing mercury in the teeth of those recruits. Yes, they were done with a quality that I could be proud of, they were done with proficiency, and they were done with the best intentions for the recruit. Today, I wonder how many people I have inadvertently poisoned in my attempt to excel in my craft. I have dedicated the rest of my life to inform those who are unaware of this toxic substance I once called my playmate.

To satisfy the flood of recruits who were training on the base for the submarine program, there were many cavities that required fillings. Dentists from all over the country were trained and convinced that the "silver" filling was the filling of choice. We didn't call it a mercury filling, even though mercury was the predominant material, containing at least 50%. The amalgam fillings were only approximately 35% silver.

While in the Navy, mercury again was a large part of my professional career. Oddly enough, during dental school, I either dozed during a lecture describing the lethal nature of mercury, or the toxic properties of this common dental filling material were not impressed upon me. All I remember learning is that when you combine 50% mercury, 35% silver, and the remaining amount in copper, tin and zinc, you create an "inert, stable filling." This was also before the AIDS epidemic, so dentists commonly performed "wet finger dentistry." We did not wear gloves or a face mask, so our exposure to mercury was at its greatest potential.

I met Captain Robert Wolcott, D.D.S. in the Navy. He had gained prominence in the dental profession regarding his research and publication on the mercury dental amalgam. He was about to retire from the Navy and accept a position as Assistant Dean and Director of Clinical Services at the prospective UCLA School of Dentistry, which was at that point only on the drawing board. He was also a friend of my previous professor at Loyola, Dr. Paul Dawson, who suggested me to be considered for a position at the dental school. During my last month of service in the Navy, Dr. Wolcott offered me a position at UCLA as Assistant Clinical Professor in the Operative Department. As part of the offer, I was asked to facilitate the development of the UCLA Dental School, which included being released from services. In 1962, I took the California State Dental Board Examination and passed. California, here I come!

So I left by myself and drove across the country to start my new career and adventure. I would go first to find a place to live. We actually thought we could buy a home using a small down payment with some savings we managed to accumulate. We had hoped to purchase our "dream home." After searching the real estate around the UCLA campus in Westwood, I found that this was out of the question. Our small savings came nowhere close to the amount of money that would be required as a deposit on a home near UCLA. However, after a few months, I sent for my family, and we rented a modest home in the San Fernando Valley. It was there that we experienced our first small earthquake and felt that we had gone through the rites of passage in becoming Californians.

So I began my teaching career, as the UCLA Dental School was in the construction stage. The staff offices were located in temporary quarters on the edge of campus referred to as the chapel. Clinical classes were held in the chemistry building where I taught a course in dental morphology - the study of the detailed anatomical structure and development of teeth. I found my work to be fascinating and enjoyable, with the exception of having to look through hundreds – yes, I did say hundreds - of extracted teeth of various anatomical forms. As part of the dental students' requirement, prior to acceptance, the student was asked to collect extracted teeth from their neighborhood dentists. These teeth were studied to determine the average anatomical configuration that could be incorporated into the wax carvings that can be transformed to plastic study models. My dexterity ability was put to a major test. The work was demanding, but rewarding. I believe these teeth are still used today.

As a young Assistant Clinical Professor, I also taught students various operative techniques, including the proper placement of dental silver-mercury fillings. Upon preparing for my first lecture, I researched the publications on this type of filling and found that, at that time, the authors of scientific literature revealed 5% of the population of this country was "allergic" to mercury. I was troubled by this statement because I was not aware of any diagnostic procedures that determined this allergy. Again, could I have missed this important fact during a dental school lecture? Figuring that 5% of 200 million is 10 million people – well, this was a sizable amount. However, later, this statement disappeared from the literature. I also soon disregarded this information and continued with the mainstream idea that mercury fillings were safe. I still have those original lecture notes from 1963.

One of the most exciting duties that I recall was conducting ergonomic research for the proposed dental clinic. Our previous

Navy research became the basis of the development of the program on efficient utilization of auxiliary personnel and the efficient placement of the evolving dental equipment in the development of the UCLA Dental Clinic. This resulted in many of the leading dental manufacturers visiting the newly developing school to present their products and latest advancements in dentistry.

An important task we were faced with was the selection of the turbine driven hand-piece. They were still in the stages of developing the efficiency of the miniature turbines used to rotate the dental drill so that they would give sufficient torque, and would not stall with low pressure. Therefore, the electronic-driven handpieces were selected which had torque, and seem to offer efficiency and advantages by reducing the size and weight of the cords required to operate the air driven handpieces. In addition, large, costly, and noisy air compressors could be avoided. However, in time, the turbine driven handpiece improved their performance and were selected for the clinics. They are still being utilized today.

During the course of developing programs for the efficient use of dental assistants, I decided to hire a head surgical nurse from the neurosurgery department to refine our efficiency studies. She had been assisting on the delicate auditory operations in the medical center. I had become acquainted with the procedures on small audio tumors which utilized many of the instruments that had been used in dentistry. I had the good fortune of observing these procedures in the neurosurgery rooms and was impressed at the sophistication and efficiencies employed by the physician and the surgical nurse. I felt that these techniques could be incorporated and developed into what is now called "four-handed dentistry."

My research in ergonomics at UCLA included the study of light - what were the ideal lighting conditions necessary for optimal working efficiency in the operatories? This required that I go to various dental offices in the area and determine the intensity and color of the operating room light. One of the offices that allowed me to carry out my study was that of another dentist, who had just completed an unusual design in his office in which he had designed, manufactured, and placed lighting that would come from the chair. His office was impressive. He offered to rent his dental office to me to start my own private practice. I accepted his offer. And so began my 50 years of private practice.

Chapter 3

Private Practice – My Dream Office

For almost ten years, I maintained a dental office on Wilshire Boulevard in Santa Monica, after renting a dental office for a brief period. We grew and thrived in Santa Monica. I maintained my position with UCLA while growing my own dental practice. However, I still wanted to build out my "dream office."

While teaching at UCLA, we also performed studies about ergonomics and improving efficiencies in dentistry. It was found that creating circles of movement and design in a dental operatory setting were ideal. The UCLA Dental School collaborated with the UCLA School of Architecture to design a workspace around the needs of the dental team. After ten years of study, the "Cognitron" was developed.

"Cognitron" was the name given to a dental service environment that divided the work space into semicircular workrooms and included storage. It was a modular unit that supplied electricity, water, air and gas from a single hole in the floor to the dual operatories and a sterilization area. The unit was a self-contained fiberglass structure that offered savings to the dentist by sharing various pieces of equipment that were housed in the central core, such as the x-ray head.

When developing a dental office space, one of the considerations a dentist has is the walls and plumbing, which can be very costly to build out. These leasehold improvements also cannot be removed by the dentist to go to another location. The Cognitron is a removable workspace and operatory that saves space and may be moved to another office. However, the most significant advantages are in providing the dental team with convenient access to the various instruments required to perform the dental services.

I was granted patents for the "Cognitron" but never went into manufacturing. I decided at the time to further research and utilize this device in my new office in Westwood, across from the UCLA campus.

In 1973, I signed a lease for office space that overlooked the UCLA campus, and enthusiastically built out the dental office utilizing the findings from our research in ergonomics. We installed the Cognitron, which served me for over 40 years. My dental practice remained in that building until 2014.

An important ingredient in developing an ergonomically designed dental office is the selection of color. After consulting with Eileen Greene, a color design expert, and some UCLA staff psychologists, it was determined that the earth tone colors where a preferable selection in order to create an environment that was more conducive to relaxation. Sharp corners and stark colors - especially red - were avoided. Instead curves and earth tones were utilized wherever possible. The curved walls and soft ambient lighting provided an atmosphere of calmness and healing. In evaluating the site and setting of the operatories, the semi-circle also offered the operating team more efficient access to the instruments and supplies.

Many UCLA staff and board members came to see my office, since it was considered a showcase for the research findings by the dental school. Representatives of dental equipment manufacturers often visited to see our latest developments in efficient dental operations in a live setting.

I continued to develop improvements in dental equipment and would often build "prototypes" for use in my own operatory. One such development was in response to the transition of stand-up dentistry to sit-down dentistry. I had created a delivery system that encapsulated the various handpieces, including drills, water spray and suction devices. I developed this for my own use. It greatly improved the efficiency of the use of the handpieces. One of the dental equipment representatives reported what he had seen in my office to his company, and as a result, version of this equipment is now used in almost every dental operatory in the country. I was never given any credit or compensation for my idea.

Another situation occurred when an ophthalmologist in my previous building, who was also my patient, noticed that I was using a dual magnifying glass while working on patients. I wore a head loupe, which is a band around my head that included a pair of magnifying glasses, side by side, extended on an 8-inch metal arm. Using this helped to improve my field of vision and precision in procedures. While discussing this apparatus, we came to the conclusion that it would be better to have jeweler scopes attached to the front of eyeglasses. So he built me a pair. While teaching courses at UCLA, numerous people inquired about where I got these special glasses. Eventually, some companies started to manufacture exactly what we created – eyeglasses with magnifying scopes attached, specifically for the dental profession, now called loupes. Personally, I would never go to a dentist that didn't use them.

Besides my work in developing better tools in dentistry, I also endeavored to learn more about overall health. The evolution in my career was now looking at causes of dental disease, in addition to restoring teeth. I was becoming somewhat aware that mercury fillings may be an issue, but I was now focusing on prevention of decay and other oral conditions.

With many of my patients in the entertainment industry, it provided me with opportunities to appear in the media regarding my philosophies about nutrition and dentistry. I also was exploring the psychological aspects of treating dental patients, using biofeedback, hypnotherapy, and other relaxation methods.

I even appeared on the Merv Griffin Show, discussing modern dental techniques and prevention. You can still see that episode on my Youtube channel, which also contains videos of several of my other appearances in the 1980s.

Many of my patients decided to join me on my quest for optimal health. Our office included a lecture room, where we discussed various "New Age" philosophies in better nutrition, exercise, and wellness. We transformed the dental office into a health center and included services like nutritional counseling, aroma therapy, iridology, massage therapy, electro-acupuncture, and other alternative therapies. In the late 1970s, this concept was ahead of its time in a dental office.

Having grown up in a small Midwestern town, it was my dream when I moved to California to have a dental practice that would take care of the biggest celebrities in Tinsel Town. Due to my affiliation with UCLA and the ability to successfully perform full-mouth restorations, some of the biggest names in show business occupied my dental chairs. While I am not at liberty to name names, since some are still patients coming to my office, I have had the unique opportunity to see inside the mouths and psyche of well-known people, of whom most people only see the outside.

There were some celebrities that would leave their ego in the waiting room, and others that needed to prove that they were "special" and didn't need to respect the doctor-patient relationship. I found the best way to deal with that situation was to show compassion, and not treat them differently than anyone else. If they didn't respect my staff or our policies, we had a saying, "Perhaps this is not the office for you." In almost every instance, they would behave respectfully once they realized that we were willing to refuse service.

Some of these celebrities became my friends. None of them were ever treated any differently than any other patient. I believe that they respected this. I have always had my patients' best interests at heart and wanted to do everything I could to help them on their journey to better health and overall wellness.

Chapter 4

Evolution of a Dentist: Allopathic to Biological to Holistic

From the start of my tenure at UCLA until 1973, I was sharing my time between teaching and developing my own dental practice. Eventually my practice grew, and I devoted full time to my private practice. In my Santa Monica office, I had been specializing in full-mouth restorations, which included removing mercury fillings. I also had been placing them, complying with the mainstream, and not questioning the possible toxic effects.

However, my interest in dentistry was moving towards the prevention of dental disease, and I was exploring the possibility of conditions of the mouth being connected to the rest of the body. My focus was on nutrition and how the mind influences overall health. I was attending seminars about various health topics, so I could learn more about incorporating good dentistry with good health habits. I wanted to pass this information on to my patients.

When I built the Westwood office, I did place an amalgamator – a device that mixes mercury with the mixed metal alloy – but it was never used. My practice had shifted into larger cases, and I had become an expert in gold work. Mercury fillings didn't really fit in with the work I was doing. I was removing mercury with no safety protocols in place.

My first experience with a patient regarding the toxic effects of mercury amalgam fillings occurred around 1970, when a new patient was referred to me with a complaint of consistent, numerous oral herpes simplex (commonly called cold sores or fever blisters). She was in her mid-forties at the time, and said that she had these lesions for the last twenty years. She suffered from them on a constant basis. If you have ever had a single cold sore in your mouth, you can have empathy for this lady who had a number of them all the time.

She was treated by various medical doctors who concluded that her condition was due to stress. One non-medical person told her that her condition may be responding to the mercury fillings in her mouth. When she presented this idea to me, I snickered to myself and told her there was no such evidence that the mercury in her fillings caused her condition. I was reluctant to remove "perfectly good fillings."

A tear rolled down her cheek. She expressed her frustration and shared with me that her husband had left her as a result of these painful ulcerations she experienced for most of her adult life. She told me that she was determined to have her "silver" fillings removed from her mouth as it was the last resort. If I did not, she said she would find someone who would. These fillings appeared to be intact and serving their original purpose, and I did not feel they required removal. However, I was concerned for her situation. I told her that I would remove the fillings for her and replace them with white composite fillings. I informed her they were less reliable. During the 1970s, composite fillings were not as refined or improved as they are today.

Approximately one month after I replaced her fillings, she sent me a letter. She thanked me for removing the fillings and said the ulcers had disappeared. I was happy for her; however, I was suspicious that the result was psychological rather than directly due to the mercury – a placebo effect. I thought perhaps her strong belief that the fillings were the cause relieved her of the ulcers. I was still not yet convinced that the mercury was causing her difficulty.

Leukemia condition affected by Mercury amalgams?

A short time later, another woman came to me with her 13-year-old daughter. She had heard that the mercury in her daughter's mouth could be contributing to her blood condition. She had been diagnosed with leukemia and was being treated at the UCLA Medical School. I told her that there was no evidence linking her condition to the fillings. Although, I did tell her that I had recently had a similar request. After more discussion, I agreed to remove her daughter's mercury fillings. I felt concern, since I had a daughter her age, who also had mercury fillings in her mouth.

Not long after, I received a phone call from the girl's oncologist at UCLA. I initially thought that he would admonish me for the removal of the fillings. He then told me that the mother recommended that he contact me regarding the removal procedure. The oncologist said that he didn't think there was any relationship between the girl's condition and the fillings, but oddly enough, her blood condition was greatly improving. We both concurred that this was the result of her strong belief.

These events were pieces of a puzzle falling into place as time went on, and as I was growing as a dentist and as a person.

Making the connection

Throughout the first half of my dental career, there were no websites to browse through, and no chat rooms or online forums to join and discuss important topics and relay information to others in real time. If a dentist wanted up-to-date information, the only methods available were to attend dental conferences and local dental society meetings, private discussions with colleagues, or receive literature via mail, including professional journals and announcements of study groups or other types of dental meetings.

From the mid-1970s to the mid-1980s, as I learned more about nutrition and how the mind affects healing and wellness, my practice services evolved. As I previously mentioned, we had health practitioners in the office giving treatments to patients in all the latest "New Age" concepts and therapies. We educated patients about how their mouth was connected to the rest of their body and how to make better decisions about managing their health. While, I wasn't placing mercury fillings at that time, I wasn't specifically against them either. I just thought it was an inferior filling to gold.

In 1973, I attended a lecture given by Dr. Hal Huggins, DDS from Colorado, who was giving courses to physicians and dentists on his theories and techniques of balancing body chemistry through blood analysis and guided nutritional supplementation. During the question-and-answer period, I shared my experiences with removing mercury fillings and the unexpected benefits, along with suspicions about the toxic nature of the mercury filling. He shared with us that he also had heard similar ideas and was suspicious as to its possible harmful effect on the human body. At a previous international dental conference, Dr. Olympio Pinto of Brazil told Dr. Huggins about all of the research and information he had compiled about the toxicity of mercury fillings and how his research had been stopped by the National Institute of Dental Health because of his topic of study. Dr. Huggins told us that he was going to continue to research the potentially toxic consequences of using mercury fillings.

I also attended transformational seminars and retreats because of my interest in my own personal development. Some of my closest friends were colleagues at UCLA Medical School, including psychiatrists conducting innovative research about human behavior. Dr. Valerie Hunt of UCLA included me in her discussions and experiments in biofeedback. I attended seminars held by Brugh Joy, MD, of the Mayo Clinic and Johns Hopkins Hospital, who was studying cancer detection through the energy fields outside of the body. It was truly was an exciting time in the research of the human potential.

The very first time I ever heard that there was any question as to the safety of mercury amalgam fillings was at a dental convention in San Francisco in 1985. It wasn't in the convention; rather it was outside the venue. As I entered the conference, there were a handful of protestors outside with signs saying that "silver" fillings were toxic. They handed me a flyer. I took it, and kept on walking. The information on that flyer would later help me find other people who were discussing this issue of mercury amalgam safety. Soon thereafter, I read the book, *The Toxic Time Bomb*, by Sam Ziff.

During this period of "awakening," there were many dentists in different parts of the country who were all coming to the same realization and forming organizations so that they might share information. In 1978, the Holistic Dental Association (HDA) formed a small group of dentists whose goal was to create a forum for the development and sharing of health-promoting therapies. In the mid-1980s, two more organizations formed: IAOMT (International Academy of Oral Medicine & Toxicology) and IABDM (International Academy of Biological Dentistry & Medicine). All of these groups are still very active and growing today.

More dentists like Dr. Huggins, and Dr. Michael Ziff (whose father, Sam Ziff wrote the book, *The Toxic Time Bomb*), many other early pioneers began to embrace the unpopular theories and alter their practices to avoid this toxic material. Several years later, Dr. Huggins wrote the well-known book, *It's All in Your Head: Diseases Caused by Silver-Mercury Fillings* and became an outspoken activist in an effort to expose the dental mercury toxicity issue.

This evolution of dentistry is called *Biological Dentistry*, which may be defined as an idea or process of dentistry that endeavors to utilize non-toxic materials in the restoration of the mouth and focuses on the unrecognized impact that dental toxins and hidden dental infections may have on overall health.

In 1985, after reading *The Toxic Time Bomb*, I called Sam Ziff to discuss the revelations in his book about the effects of mercury in dentistry. He mentioned there was a new group that his son and other dentists were forming (IAOMT) and were going to study this well-hidden topic in a scientific manner. Their motto was, "Show Me the Science." As a UCLA educator and researcher, a scientific basis is essential for developing new treatments and materials in dentistry. In the past, I had been a staunch supporter of the use of the mercury filling. I was coming to the realization that my quest for knowledge about optimal health of the human body was about to take a turn, that would refute my dental training and education, my colleagues, and what I taught so many students over the years.

It would have been easier to do nothing, but that's not me.

Changing my perspective as a dentist

I started in my profession as a mainstream, "allopathic" dentist. Allopathic dentistry is defined as primarily dealing with the symptoms of a disease process, addressing the perfection of the preparation of the tooth and the accuracy of the fit of the dental filling, so as to prevent bacteria from reoccurring decay. A dentist's income is primarily based on the number of fillings or repairs that are done, without addressing the preventive aspect. This was the height of allopathic dentistry. Drilling, filling and billing. There was little thought or curiosity of the short or long-term impact of the procedure or dental materials on the patient's health.

There was a time in dentistry, around 1970, when dentists attempted to focus on prevention. As a result, a group of dentists assembled and found that there was no real financial return from this approach. Whether applied to dentistry or general medicine, prevention was rarely acknowledged, especially by insurance companies. Because of my personal focus of prevention in my dental practice, one of my patients, who was a top executive in the insurance industry, asked me to submit an article regarding the benefits of prevention as it relates to health and the cost of care. After insurance companies figured out it was more profitable to cover preventive care like teeth cleaning appointments, prevention became more accepted and sometimes required.

Biological dentistry to holistic dentistry

While educating myself in the bio-compatibility issues of filling materials, I felt the human body was not just about a collection of anatomical parts brilliantly working together. Logically, it also included the thought process, emotions and spiritual growth. How could a dentist treat such a sacred part of the body as the mouth and not have any effect on the whole being? I was moved to consider the whole being. I brought my dentistry to a holistic-spiritual level: the incorporation of healing with the mind, body and spirit.

My long-time friend and patient, Dick Van Dyke had encouraged me to read Andrew Weil's book, *The Natural Mind*. That book gave me the motivation to continue my study of the mind and healing. It opened my own mind to the possibility of the non-drug, non-symptom approach to health. Disease is a result of a blockage of energy. This energy that can be read and identified, and is part of the healing process.

Western medicine cannot ignore the Chinese perspective of disease; that the energy - the chi, the aura, or an electromagnetic force – can be read, seen, and electronically verified as part of the healing process. As viewed in acupuncture, the teeth are located on energy meridians and correlate to other organs in the body. Disease is a blockage of energy, and depending on which body part, genetics of the organ, the temperament and stresses of the patient, nutrition, environment – these all play a role in the manifestation of a disease, illness or malfunction that results in the lack of circulation of energy. The result may be that metabolic processes shut down, and result in a buildup of acid. Natural medicine provides methods to re-establish the flow of energy and life force. That flow of energy is connected to the mind, which has the ability to attain, direct, block, nurture and affect that flow. In a later chapter, I will explain more about the mouth's connection to and reflection of the body.

Now, you are probably saying to yourself, "Are we still talking about dentistry?" My response is, "Yes, especially dentistry." Humans are made up of complex systems: physical, mental, emotional, and spiritual. Are these systems operating independently of each other? None of us would believe that. However, in the midst of all this, I am a scientist, researcher and clinician. I wasn't going to just take someone's word for it. I bought equipment that measured electrical currents in the body, vapor measurement equipment, and anything else I could find to prove or disprove all of the hypotheses along the way. I needed to "see the needles move."

Chapter 5

Getting Sicker and Sicker

Dentistry, whether holistic or allopathic, is a very physically, mentally and emotionally demanding occupation. Dentists are in a physically difficult position – standing or sitting, leaning over the patient, and performing micro-surgery throughout the day. We are often dealing with fearful, stressed patients and a busy staff. Most of us aren't aware of the level of toxicity that resides in our dental materials and operatory. Every person reacts to these conditions differently. We all have different levels of tolerance and susceptibility. We do know that dentists have one of the highest suicide rates, that is only second to physicians. Even though I was involved with learning more about the effects of the mercury filling on patients, I somehow still didn't fully make the correlation to my own exposure and potential for illness.

My toxic burnout

Over the past five decades, I have been in contact with many chemicals and drugs that we now know may affect our body's health. Not only did I develop leg and back disorders from my physical work in dentistry, but I was also exposed to the biggest hazard of my profession – mercury, the second most deadly metal on the face of the earth, next to radioactive plutonium.

In the late 1980s, I was experiencing Chronic Fatigue Syndrome, burnout, depression, and Epstein-Barr Syndrome, to mention a few. My muscles ached, my short-term memory was affected, I had ringing in my ears, and I could not sleep. The doctors prescribed more drugs, but they only temporarily dealt with the symptoms, not the cause. Also, the drugs had undesirable side effects.

I was at my wit's end and did not think that I could continue practicing dentistry. This was a very stressful idea to contemplate. I had always thought that I was physically fit and had an exercise program consisting of weight training and jogging. However, I became too tired to continue. I got sicker and sicker. I also had a number of injuries from weight training and the trauma of the high impact on my joints from jogging. This further damaged my already weakened body.

Throughout the late 1970s and 1980s, I continued to gather more information regarding the toxic effects of mercury. During my investigation, I went through a divorce and a series of failed relationships. I found myself quite depressed. I had difficulty sleeping, cold hands and feet, and the ringing in my ears that I had endured throughout my life was intensifying. I became very sensitive to odors like cleaning products, gasoline and perfumes. I found myself becoming increasingly tired and fatigued and could no longer work a full day. I had become very irritable, to which my employees and family can attest. I was unable to witness violence on television or anything controversial. I could only tolerate watching the History Channel or nature films.

I lost weight and had a very unhealthy, emaciated appearance. My son encouraged me to join a health club so I could become more physically fit. I was accustomed to having a strong, healthy body, and thought that I could restore it to a more healthy condition. However, I still didn't have the energy to work out, especially at the end of the dentistry workday, as I continued to be exposed to more and more toxins daily.

I recall standing in the shower at the club, after a short group of exercises, and concluding that I could not continue. I felt I was getting older and breaking down, even though I was about 50 years old at the time. I thought perhaps my age and depression was responsible for my increasing weakness.

At the time, I had been doing some research on sodium alginate as a physical detoxifier of heavy metal and radiation. Shortly after the Russian Chernobyl incident, I had been invited to speak at the People's Forum at the United Nations in New York City. However, I was becoming so weak that I felt I could not make the journey. Only after strong encouragement from my colleagues did I decide to make the trip.

My ideas about mercury toxicity were based on having mercury fillings. I was managing other people's mercury issues every day. However, I had no mercury fillings in my mouth. I did not consider my own mercury exposure: playing with mercury as a child and working with mercury for decades as a practicing dentist.

During this time, prior to the AIDS epidemic, dentists did not wear gloves or protective masks. I did not realize that I was vulnerable to the colorless, odorless toxic fumes of mercury that were part of the practice of conventional, allopathic dentists at the time. When a dentist drills in the presence of mercury, the heat from the drill will produce a toxic mercury vapor that is inhaled by the patient, dental assistant, and dentist. Mercury has a half-life up to several decades and was still tenaciously clinging to the cells in my body.

Ironically, the correlation that perhaps my own mercury exposure was responsible for my steady decline in health did not occur to me. Studies have been done that reveal that the oxygen coming out of the cells of a mercury-toxic patient, like myself, was reduced by 65%. Mercury binds to oxygen-binding sites on the hemoglobin molecule where there should be oxygen. As a result, even though I was breathing enough oxygen, my body was starving for it, which contributed to my fatigue and cold extremities.

Developing one condition to fight another

I was also experiencing uncomfortable symptoms of gas and constipation. After reading several books, I thought that my condition was partially the result of yeast or Candida albicans. It was recommended that I go on a yeast-free diet, avoid sugar, take large doses of Nystatin (a synthetic form of Vitamin C), and take frequent saunas to flush toxins out. I made these changes, but my condition only improved slightly. Science has since found the yeast organism may actually be a body defense by binding mercury molecules together into a larger molecule, which is more difficult to be absorbed in the large intestines. So eliminating the Candida removed what was protecting me from the mercury.

I found that when I was constipated, I felt more ill. When I kept a clean colon, I felt better. My condition seemed to improve with colon irrigation or colonics. But I couldn't maintain the improvement because the mercury in my body was killing the natural flora in my digestive tract, allowing the pathological bacteria to reside. So I started a regimen of supplementation of the natural flora – Lactobacillus acidophilus, Bifidobacterium bifidum, and other friendly bacteria, which I continue to take today.

I still attempted the difficult task of eliminating sugar from my diet. As an adult, I was accustomed to sugar in various forms, from ice cream to Martinis. However, I could not consume any sugar or alcoholic beverages without severe headaches, bouts of hypoglycemia and intense periods of fatigue.

My health started showing some improvement, and I began to gain weight. I started to recover from the critical stage of my illness, becoming stronger with determination and support from my family. I continued exercising, colon cleansing, and avoiding foods that were irritating to my condition.

Music became a source of relief for me. I used to play Rachmaninov's 2nd and 3rd Piano Concerto over and over. I found it to be calming yet motivating and a way to distract myself from my physical condition. I also listened to motivational tapes to reinforce my determination to resolve my mysterious illness. I was in search of anything that would bring relief and resolution.

However, I was still addressing the symptoms and not the cause. I would soon come to the realization that my childhood friend, that seductive vial of mercury, was really my enemy, and the real battle was about to be fought. The frightening part was not if there was mercury in my body, but just how much.

Chapter 6

Bouncing Back - Literally

In the 1980s, I formed a study group in Los Angeles, consisting of dentists and physicians to further investigate the mercury issue. I had the good fortune to meet Hans Gruenn, MD, a German physician who regularly treated patients for heavy metal toxicity, which he said might be a major cause for many of the symptoms I had been experiencing.

At the same time, the IAOMT, in collaboration with Dr. Aposhian from the University of Arizona, conducted a study of the diagnostic and therapeutic properties of a chemical agent developed in China and Russia during the Cold War called DMPS (2,3-dimercapto-1-propane-sulfonic acid). The chemical would bind, challenge or chelate the mercury molecule from the cells of the body and release it into the circulatory system, where the toxins could be released into the fecal matter, urine, sweat and breath.

This was the first time that scientists could prove, once and for all, if mercury was actually being retained in the body. DMPS would be administered to volunteering dentists who were members of the IAOMT.

Prior to this time, conventional blood, urine, and fecal tests revealed no elevated mercury without first administering a disclosing agent. Mercury concentrates in fatty tissues, especially in the brain, which is made mostly of fat. Blood tests aren't an accurate measurement of total body burden of mercury.

Our newly formed group developed our own study, and I was one of the members who volunteered to participate in the DMPS study. Dr. Gruenn administered the DMPS in our group. The results clearly showed that I released a large amount of mercury. Other dentists also released mercury but not as much as I had, which was described as "industrial levels" of toxicity. On my lab report, the level of mercury was literally off of the chart. There wasn't enough paper to show the full amount on the graph. This truly alarmed me. I had thought my natural program had been enough to deal with the level of mercury that I suspected was present. I was feeling better, but, nonetheless, I had extremely high amounts of mercury still in my body. I wondered what the test result would have revealed in the beginning, before I started any health regimen.

In the past, the American Dental Association tested volunteers at a convention, but only took blood samples. They did not challenge the blood test with the disclosing agents, such as DMPS. Therefore, they concluded that mercury was not an issue; for if it were, dentists should have more than the general public. Recent tests have shown that dentists do have more mercury than the general population, and dental assistants have a greater threat, since they are the ones who mix the alloy and mercury.

Over the next twenty years, I studied natural methods, using certain foods along with chelating agents to detoxify the body. I discovered that mercury, as an example, is very difficult to diagnose and treat because it resides in the cells of certain tissues and is not ordinarily found in blood or urine, which are the common laboratory tests prescribed by most physicians to diagnose illness.

I also found that most toxins, when dislodged from inside certain cells, will be released in bowel movements, and a smaller amount in urine and sweat. I had always been constipated and too tired to work up a sweat and was not a great fan of drinking water. It became apparent why I had gotten sicker and sicker. I was not releasing the toxins fast enough and was continuing to take more into my body. Mercury in the brain and central nervous system has a considerably longer half-life than in the rest of the body, which can be years and decades. Therefore, the mercury that I had absorbed over several decades was still present. This new information was enlightening, but I knew it also held difficult challenges for me.

During my release of mercury, I was revisited with more severe symptoms. When mercury is released in the body and goes into the circulatory system, it crosses the blood-brain barrier, and some of the symptoms can return. I continued to use the DMPS challenge as a means of detoxifying and monitoring progress, along with natural methods, including diet. It was also very important that this was all done under a doctor's care. It is essential that any detoxification program be supervised by a qualified health care professional.

My task was to facilitate detoxification by eating foods that naturally remove the toxins that I had been accumulating. This included garlic, chlorella, cilantro, parsley, spirulina, and others. I also avoided the foods that contained mercury, like certain fish (tuna has the highest levels), sushi, and vegetables that have been sprayed with the pesticides containing mercury. By the way, the safest fish to eat is wild salmon or halibut.

Bouncing back to health

I attended a lecture in Seattle on detoxification of mercury through DMPS and DMSA, which were used to chelate or challenge the mercury hiding in the fatty tissue of the body. The lecturer said the most effective exercise to encourage the release of mercury was a mini-trampoline, also known as a rebounder. I liked the idea because I was spending too much time at the health club and wanted to exercise at home.

As soon as I returned, I went to the local sporting goods store and purchased an inexpensive, circular rebounder. Although the rebounder was of low quality with poor springs and a hard bounce, I was determined to improve my health. So up and down on the rebounder I went.

Much of the toxins will reside or pass through the lymphatic system throughout the body. This system has no pump and relies on body movement to transport the toxins out of the cells and to bring the nutrients into the cells. The lymphatic pump becomes very active during rebound exercise, often increasing lymph flow 10 to 30 fold. I found that bouncing on a mini-trampoline considerably improved this circulation. Consequently, a mini-trampoline or rebounder became a daily routine in my life.

Slowly, after months of dieting, cleansing the body and rebound exercise, I began to get better. A laboratory test that was administrated by Dr. Gruenn showed that I was eliminating those life-threatening toxins. I found rebounding to be the most effective and proactive physical activity in my recovery.

When I first started bouncing, I proceeded very slowly because I had a football injury to my knee. I was able to safely use the rebounder with my injury when I added a system of support consisting of straps hanging from an overhead bar, like a chin-up bar. My initial three-minute workouts while nursing my knee evolved into longer workouts without pain while being able to achieve an aerobic state. I placed the rebounder in my large, walk-in closet, along with an oxygen tank. Occasionally, I would exercise while wearing an oxygen mask.

The distressing symptoms I previously experienced – cold hands, ringing in the ears, insomnia, etc. – were improving, to my delight. I was feeling better each day. Bouncing on the rebounder became a part of my daily routine. If I missed a day, I didn't feel as well that day. My health continued to improve, and I became stronger.

I could only take so much time out during the day to exercise, and I wanted to use my time as efficiently as possible. Throughout my career, I was always looking for better, more efficient ways to work or modify equipment to increase productivity and efficiency. Re-evaluating my method of exercise was no different.

The rebounder I was using was small, round, and had a firm bounce. I went through a lot of rebounders – the springs would break or the mat would tear. So I started designing a better system of rebound exercise. I created a rebounder in the shape of a trapezoid. This modification added more jumping surface area and was more flexible with larger springs and a high-quality mat, giving it a softer bounce. I also wanted to work on my upper body while getting aerobic exercise, so I added an overhead strength training system in my closet doorway. I could develop my upper body while I bounced on the rebounder.

It was the unique combination of aerobics, strength training, and cell detoxification that enabled me to see the most dramatic changes in my body. I called it "Bouncercise®."

They say necessity is the mother of invention. I needed Bouncercise, and it became an important component in my recovery. Many of my patients noticed my transformation and inquired about the reason for my success. I introduced my program to them, and they soon began to improve their health. It has been especially welcomed by seniors, disabled persons, and other people who previously felt unstable on a rebounder.

For the benefits of Bouncercise to be shared by everyone, I developed and patented The Freedom Spring System®. Yes, this may be viewed as a shameless plug for an exercise system that is on the market today. But I felt compelled to share what I had developed with my colleagues and patients. At the age of 81, I still

Bouncercise most every day, including throughout my recent health challenges, which I will talk about in a later chapter.

My personal life and career have been about learning how to take responsibility and control of my own health, to keep an open mind and to come up with better ideas whenever possible. I feel strongly that had I not gone down the "alternative" path, my dental career would have been much shorter, and perhaps my life, too.

Chapter 7

Mercury in Dentistry

The use of mercury in dentistry is an extremely complex and controversial topic. When dental mercury is the subject of an online news article or blog post, it is often a lengthy, heated debate. For the purposes of my story, I will share with you my experiences, findings, and realizations as a dentist, scientist, and hopeful human being regarding the dental mercury issue. In simplistic terms, I will cover some important points that may help people, including dentists and consumers, understand mercury's place in dentistry.

Mercury, it's a thing

Let's start with acknowledging mercury itself. The symbol for mercury on the periodic table is Hg, coming from its Greek name, hydrargyrum. Aristotle, in 400 BC, described it as "liquid silver" due to its mobility and shiny surface.

Mercury is one of two metals that is liquid at room temperature. The other is Bromine. Because of this mobile state, mercury is also known as quicksilver. At room temperature, mercury is constantly vaporizing.

Mercury and all of its compounds are toxic. Mercury can be absorbed through the skin and mucous membranes, and mercury vapors can be inhaled. Other toxic forms of mercury are its organic compounds, such as dimethyl mercury and methylmercury. On a scale of 1 to 10, in terms of toxicity of all the elements on the periodic table, mercury is a solid 10. It is only second to radioactive elements, like plutonium, in terms of lethality. All forms of mercury are extremely dangerous. None are "inert" or safe, and exposure to all should be avoided.

Mercury in dentistry: a love story

It is important to mention the history of mercury fillings because what happened in the 1800s really set the tone for the course for future events.

Before people were trained as dentists, the local barber often pulled teeth, using gold, lead plugs or melted coins to make dental fillings. By the 1820s, dentistry, as a profession, was in its early stages. The first dental school opened in 1828 in Baltimore. The first local dental organization was formed in New York in 1834. From that group, the first national organization, called the American Society of Dental Surgeons (ASDS), was formed in 1840.

The use of mercury in fillings began in the United States in 1833. Edward Crawcour and his nephew, Moses Crawcour, came from a transient Polish family of dentists that lived in England. The Crawcours used an amalgam mixture called "silver paste" that was named and invented by a French dentist, Auguste Taveau. This paste was made from filings of the French franc, which contained silver, copper, and tin, then mixed with mercury. The Crawcour family placed fillings throughout England, claiming to have been dentists for European royal families.

Edward and Moses Crawcour came to America, traveled around, set up in hotel parlors and charged wealthy patrons large fees for dentistry. They called it Royal Mineral Succedaneum, which was another deceptive name for the mercury amalgam dental filling. They would plug the patient's cavity with the amalgam without first removing the decay – and called it painless dentistry. The Crawcours' business initially was quite successful, and greatly affected the incomes of local, ethical dental practitioners. However, eventually, the poor dentistry produced loose fillings, broken and discolored teeth, due to the expansion of the cheap amalgam. The Crawcours made a quick exit back to England.

It is said that six dentists got together, pooled their money, and had a filling placed by one of the Crawcours. The dentists then removed its contents and had it analyzed by a chemist, who identified the mercury mixed in with the other metals. They found the new mercury amalgam was cheap and easy to use, and felt that if used properly with good dentistry, it could be a viable filling material.

In 1843, the ASDS stated that "the use of amalgam constitutes malpractice." Dentists who did use mercury amalgam were considered quacks. In 1844, it was noted in the American Journal of Dental Science that the bad effects of mercury on the body preclude use of the dental amalgam in any case. Members were forced to sign a pledge that they would not use the mercury amalgam or they would be expelled from membership.

Some dentists didn't have sufficient skills to use the alternate filling of gold in all cases, and gold was much more expensive than the mercury alternative. The ASDS was quite harsh about compliance with the pledge and even visited dentists' offices to see if they were using the mercury amalgam. Eventually, the ASDS reluctantly rescinded its pledge, but due to declining membership, it folded in 1856. One dentist commented in a dental journal of the time, that perhaps if the organization had come up with an alternative, it could have survived. Just as today, money is often more important than health and safety.

After the dissolution of the ASDS, another organization called the American Dental Convention quickly formed in its place in 1856. This organization had no requirements about the use of dental amalgam; it was only necessary to be a dentist. This group eventually gave way to the American Dental Association, which was established in 1859. The Southern Dental Association, which had broken away from national groups, formed during the Civil War Era, merged with the American Dental Association and became the National Dental Association. It was then renamed the American Dental Association in 1922.

The American Dental Association (ADA) calls this period, "The First Amalgam War," beginning with the 1833 arrival of the Crawcours, and ending with the folding of the ASDS in 1856. Had the dentists at the time accepted the ban of mercury in dentistry, it is quite possible that the ASDS would be in existence today, and mercury would not be considered a dental material.

At the turn of the 20th Century, homeopathic physicians spoke up against the use of dental amalgam. As seen in medical literature at that time, they claimed the body absorbed the mercury, threw the "system out of balance" and caused "derangement of the spleen, stomach, liver, kidneys, nerves, mucous membranes, the skin, etc." The standard response of the dental community was that "people with amalgam fillings were as healthy as any other persons." It is the same response today.

The Second Amalgam War started in 1926, when Alfred E. Stock, a leading chemist at the Kaiser Wilhelm Institute in Germany declared the dental amalgam a "nasty sin against humanity." He stated that mercury fillings should be removed if a physician could find no other cause for neurological disorders or inflammation of the mucous membrane, especially of the respiratory tract. However, in 1931, the National Bureau of Standards in Washington DC concurred with the dental community and declared that mercury poisoning from dental amalgams was not justified. After being discredited by the ADA and with most of his work destroyed in the bombings of World War II, Dr. Stock became discouraged. Thus ended the Second Amalgam War. Dr. Stock later died from mercury poisoning as a result of his research.

There were many reports of diseases that were associated with the use of mercury in dentistry. However, even though they are reported in a historical sense, they are dismissed as coincidence or probably caused by some other factor. Where was the concern, diligent investigation, research, or even curiosity by the dental community? The love affair of the mercury filling by the American Dental Association reads like a drugstore paperback novel about a clingy girlfriend with a cruel boyfriend.

The Third Amalgam War is currently in full swing. It began in 1973, when several dentists around the country began questioning the safety of the mercury filling. This time, with the concerted efforts of organizations like IAOMT, IABDM, HDA, Consumers for Dental Choice, Dental Amalgam Mercury Syndrome (DAMS), TALKInternational.com, and injured consumers and dental personnel, there will be no giving up until mercury is removed from dentistry and protocols are in place for safe removal. As they say, the third time is the charm.

Mercury in the dental office

Typical mercury fillings contain approximately 50% mercury. The rest of the filling is usually made up of an alloy of silver, zinc, copper, and tin. It is very misleading to call it a "silver filling." It sounds so much more palatable, doesn't it? According to a 2014 Zogby Poll, 57% of consumers are not aware that there is any mercury in dental fillings, and only 11% reported being told by their dentists that "amalgam" fillings are mostly mercury.

When a dentist orders mercury amalgam from the dental supplier, the elemental mercury comes in capsules, along with the alloy. Before it is placed on the tooth, it is first shaken by an amalgamator for mixing. This process is called trituration, which is the mechanical mixing of the alloy and mercury. In the past, trituration was also done by hand using a mortar and pestle. The amalgam filling was then put in a squeeze cloth to extract the extra mercury. This was a very toxic scenario, with exposure to elemental and vaporized mercury, which I performed many times.

The invention of the capsules and electronic mixer has decreased mercury exposure, but not enough. Since mixing the mercury amalgam is usually performed by the dental assistant, they are particularly exposed to mercury vapors.

Reading the manufacturer warnings is really very disturbing, since this is a substance that we are putting just a couple inches from a child's brain, and perhaps yours, too.

Here are some of the highlights of warnings of amalgam fillings as stated on the 14-page Material Safety Data Sheet for Aristaloy Fillings, dated 8/11/2014, available through one of the largest dental supply companies in America, Henry Schein Dental:

Hazard(s) Identification:
- Very toxic
- Very toxic by inhalation
- Toxic
- May Cause harm to unborn child. Toxic: danger of serious damage to health by prolonged exposure through inhalation

NFPA Rating: Health = 4 (extreme health hazard, lethal or deadly)
HMIS Rating: Health = *4, (Life-threatening, major or permanent damage may result from single or repeated exposures. Asterisk denotes chronic hazard, Long-term exposure to the material could cause a health problem.)

Composition/information on ingredients:
- Dangerous components: 50% mercury

Environmental Precautions and Disposal Considerations:
- Do not allow product to reach sewage system or any water course.
- Inform respective authorities in case of seepage into water course or sewage system.

Transport Information:
Danger Code (Kemler): 80 (corrosive or slightly corrosive substance)

There are 14 pages of warnings. I doubt that most dentists leave that in their waiting room for recreational reading just before they implant it into the patient's mouth, and most aren't telling their patients about the warnings.

The ADA stands by the safety of mercury fillings. On the ADA consumer website, www.mouthhealthy.org, they state, "It's important to know that when combined with the other metals, it forms a safe, stable material."

Studies have shown that under the conditions of infections associated with dental amalgams, methylmercury is generated in the mouth. According to the USGS (US Geological Survey), "Methylmercury is the form most readily incorporated into biological tissues and most toxic to humans."

The manufacturer warns of how toxic the product is before it goes in the mouth, and it also gives safety precautions for disposal, including a statement that the product should never reach a sewage system. How is it safe IN someone's mouth? It's okay to be in your mouth but not your sewer?

For most people, that is all they need to hear before they say, "I think I'll opt for the white filling." It doesn't take a degree in science to see the problem with mercury fillings.

There is a wealth of information available about the toxicity of dental amalgam fillings. There is no debate that mercury is toxic. It's a fact. As we continue in this book, you will find more information about the safety and toxicity of dental mercury. I will also provide a list of in the Recommended Resources if you need more detailed information.

Mercury filling removal – Do no harm

Today, many people choose to have composite (tooth-colored) fillings without any awareness about the hazards of mercury fillings. They are often choosing composites because they look better, not because they were consciously making a healthier choice. However, if they are having a mercury filling replaced, they are not likely to be aware of the hazards involved in removing the old, dark toxic filling. And if they go to a dentist who isn't aware or chooses ignorance about this hazardous situation, they are both putting themselves at great risk.

If there is one thing I could impress upon the public most regarding mercury fillings, it would be to make sure the dentist who is removing the mercury filling is protecting the patient, himself and his staff. When a dentist removes the filling with the high speed drill, the heat of the drill on the mercury is creating mercury vapors, the most toxic form of mercury. Without protection, the patient, dentist, and dental assistant are all breathing these toxic vapors.

The IAOMT has developed protocols for safe mercury removal. These protocols are constantly being reviewed and updated. It would be wise for any person who is considering having mercury fillings removed to ask their dentist what precautions they use to protect the patient from mercury during the procedure.

Even among biological dentists, you will see varying degrees of protection and different types of equipment. Some dentists use full body suits and gas masks to protect themselves and the assistant. No matter the degree your dentist "suits up," I believe that most of the biological dentists go to great lengths to protect the patient.

Patient protection during safe mercury removal consists of giving the patient their own filtered air or oxygen source so they are not breathing in the mercury vapors. Full body and face covering for the patient, including eyewear should also be used. The procedure itself should include the use of high volume evacuation and copious amounts of water to keep the area as cool as possible. Be sure to visit the IAOMT.org website for the latest protocols suggested for your safety.

If your dentist is concerned about your safety and is using the safety protocols for mercury removal, the staff should be able to tell you over the telephone what precautions are used. If they don't know what you are talking about, then find another dentist.

Mercury fillings, dental insurance, and the poverty factor

Many dental insurance companies will fully cover mercury fillings for cavities in back teeth, while restricting coverage for composite fillings. So if you need a filling on a molar tooth, and you want your dental insurance to fully cover your dental work, you will have to opt for the mercury filling. Many people, unaware of the toxicity issues, will choose the mercury filling so they don't have to pay more out of pocket. Fillings should be a decision for consumers and their dentists – not an insurance company.

Another problem is free or low-cost dental services to people in low-income families, military personnel, prisoners, people with disabilities and minorities are still subjected to amalgam. These services often don't inform the patient that a composite filling may be available upon request. The default filling material used is the mercury filling.

I remember a new patient who came to me several years ago. He was a disabled Gulf War veteran, who had previously come to one of my lectures about the dangers of mercury fillings. During the diagnosis at his appointment, he told me that if he was to go to the Veterans Administration dentist to have his mercury fillings replaced, his teeth would be refilled with mercury. He was not given a choice. He was living on his Veterans Benefits and could not afford to have the work done in a private dental office. He seemed like such a caring person and had sacrificed his own health and safety while serving our country. I couldn't bear the thought of him being placed in jeopardy again, so I replaced his fillings pro bono. There were times throughout my dental career when I felt I needed to pay it forward and have been blessed to be given the opportunity to do so.

Our governmental agencies, including dental boards, and insurance companies need to re-evaluate the real costs of placing and unsafely removing mercury fillings. They should ensure that people are not being implanted with something that may affect their overall health over the long term.

Dental mercury pollution

According to the EPA, "approximately 50 percent of mercury entering local waste treatment plants comes from dental amalgam waste." They further state that "mercury released through amalgam discharges can be easily managed and prevented." A responsible dentist will use an amalgam separator in their office.

An amalgam separator is a device designed to remove amalgam waste particles from dental office wastewater. When a dental office does not use an amalgam separator, particles containing mercury can be suctioned into the dental unit vacuum line and discharged into the public sewer system. As previously mentioned, the Material Safety Data Sheet for dental amalgam specifically states,

"Do not allow product to reach sewage system or any water course."

The ADA recently spent $2.8 million to fight the EPA ruling on dental amalgam separators. The ADA is the third-highest-spending health professionals' lobby. After pressure from consumer groups like Consumers for Dental Choice and the findings of the EPA itself, negotiations with the ADA resulted in a voluntary program in 2007 for use of amalgam separators by dentists. Since then, it has been found that only 2% of dentists actually placed the separators in their office, in unregulated areas. There are now eleven states that have mandatory amalgam separator laws, but it is estimated that only about 60 to 65% of dentists comply.

Amalgam separators cost an average of approximately $700 annually. With dentists being such a significant source of mercury pollution, why isn't this just considered a cost of doing business and being responsible for the protection of the environment from their own actions? One would think that a professional organization like the ADA would want their members to act responsibly toward the environment. Finally, in 2007, the ADA suggested the use of amalgam separators in their Best Management Practices, but they oppose mandatory laws.

Crematoriums are also part of the discussion of mercury pollution. An average cremation releases 2 to 4 grams of mercury into the environment. When people are cremated, the mercury dental fillings are vaporized. After entering the air and then falling in rain, it becomes concentrated in fish and, if eaten during pregnancy, can cause harm to unborn children. It has been estimated that crematoriums release approximately 2.5 - 3 tons of mercury air pollution each year in the United States, which is attributed to mercury fillings.

Recently, the United Nations, through The Minamata Convention on Mercury, passed a global treaty to protect human health and the environment from the adverse effects of mercury, including consumer products like the mercury dental filling. The ADA and the IAOMT were involved in those negotiations, along with consumer groups, including Consumers for Dental Choice and the World Alliance for Mercury-Free Dentistry.

Here is the ADA's position at the negotiations: "We urge the United States to oppose any effort in these negotiations to ban or limit the availability of dental amalgam." The ADA also states that dental office mercury is only 1% of the total sources of mercury entering the environment, which is a misleading statistic when you consider that dental offices account for 50% of all the mercury coming into the water treatment plants. Why not stop it at the source?

Okay, Mercury is bad. What is the perfect filling material?

There is no 100% safe filling. There is no substitute for a healthy tooth. All restorative dentistry is a compromise. The optimal dental care is prevention.

Dentistry, however, has gone far beyond any other branch of medicine in designing body parts for replacement. Dental restorations function in a very efficient manner, as opposed to other body parts that have been replaced. Dental restorations are a compromise. The disease process or decay of the tooth is brought on by acid, which is coming from a number of places, such as bacteria in the mouth from lack of brushing, and acid originating in the body, and consuming products containing acid.

For the erosion of the teeth, there are basically three filling materials available: mercury amalgam, composite and gold. Gold has always been a favorable filling material, although it requires sharp technical skills and is clearly more expensive. From the standpoint of longevity, I can tell you that the gold filling restoration in my mouth has been there for at least 40 years. Is it a compromise? I believe that one must evaluate the effectiveness of a restoration. It is understood that it replaces the tooth structure. However, is it generating problems in other areas of the body? We will explore the impact of dentistry on the rest of the body in a later chapter.

The materials that we are using to replace the amalgam fillings are petroleum-based products, the resins. The coloring obtained, and the cements, and fabrication materials used consist of silica – which are binding agents. They are in the benzene and petroleum-based families, which can be toxic. A dentist needs to seek out non-BPA composite material – which is now available. BPA is an endocrine disruptor and a factor in cancer. Some composite resins are not as durable, but the advantages lie in that when they are properly administered, they will cling to the tooth structure, requiring minimal removal of healthy tooth.

A word about costs and longevity

A common statement about composite fillings is that they are more expensive than mercury amalgam fillings and don't last as long. I would disagree with that statement. In terms of materials, the main variables are that it may take a dentist longer to place a composite filling and require a greater degree of skill to reduce sensitivity. The dentist also needs to purchase more materials for the placement of composite fillings, such as bonding agents, varnish solution, and various shades of the composite materials in order to match the color of the tooth.

One of the differences in the preparation of the filling is that the composite filling will bind to the tooth. As a result, less tooth structure will need to be removed than for a mercury filling, which is placed mechanically by dovetails and ledges. The amalgam filling requires carving out more angles and taking away more of the tooth. Mercury fillings are a lot easier to place, but they are not a better filling. Mercury fillings may weaken the teeth, which makes them more susceptible to breaking. Broken teeth are very expensive to restore.

According to a study entitled, "A 24-month evaluation of amalgam and resin-based composite restorations," it was found that both filling materials have similar longevity factors. One important difference with the amalgam filling is that it may eventually act as a wedge and split the tooth. In addition, due to the density of the mercury filling, an x-ray won't show decay around the filling. As a result, a person is likely to have the mercury filling longer than they should and may experience tooth loss or root canal because of the undetected weakening of the tooth.

Composite materials have improved and can now last as long as a mercury filling. Some manufacturers of composite fillings continue to develop filling materials while considering toxic effects. In terms of mechanical and restorative benefits and toxicity, the composite filling far outweighs the cost savings and risks of the mercury filling.

Progress - slow, but sure

It is interesting that some of the greatest strides in the anti-mercury dental filling movement in recent years has come through environmental strategies. What does that say about our concern about our health as a country? Actually, I believe it says more about the power of money, the undue influence over governmental agencies by the corporations that those agencies are supposed to be regulating, and the ability to control a national conversation.

Chapter 8

Why Don't Dentists Know This?

Quite frankly, my colleagues and I are astounded that dental mercury is still being used. In the 1980s, we were sure that in ten years, mercury would no longer be used as a filling material. Here it is, 2015, and the ADA is still controlling the narrative on the safety of dental mercury.

It is not my intention to blame or point fingers at any particular group or individual. I don't believe that is how to effect change. However, when a reasonable person reviews the evidence and sees misleading information that has been given to the government and the public for over 100 years, it is very difficult to not get upset. It is, therefore, with great restraint and understanding that I delicately move forward.

A frequently asked question

At most lectures that I have given, a person stands up at the end and asks, "Why don't dentists know this?" It is an excellent question.

I admit that I was part of the problem. In lectures, I told my UCLA students that when mercury is combined with an alloy, it is "inert." I told them that because I was told the same thing. It wasn't questioned. I didn't know that the dental profession was in a long-term denial of the toxic effects of mercury fillings, including the mercury vapors that came from the filling after it was placed.

I also told my students that 5% of the population is allergic to mercury. This was the information that I repeated from my own education. But think about that number. Do the math. In 1965, the population of the United States was 194 million people; that would make 9,700,000 people with allergic reactions to mercury fillings!

The ADA kept changing the number of people that are likely to be allergic to mercury fillings. After it was pointed out to them in 1984 (likely by Dr. Hal Huggins), that a number like that would be considered an epidemic in epidemiological terms, they quickly changed the number to 1%. Then in 1989, it was changed to 1 in 1 million, and then back up to 3% in 1991. Presently, the ADA claims that less than 1% of the population is "allergic" to mercury fillings, or that it is very rare. They claim to be a scientifically driven organization but show no scientific basis for this information.

Where do they get this statistic regarding the amount of people that are allergic to mercury? Are they referring to a particular study? If so, hopefully, they will someday point to the source of their data. Studies about mercury allergy do exist. For example, studies on dental students were performed in 1976 and 1985, and they revealed up to 32% and 26% of students had mercury allergies, respectively.

Also, how does someone know if they are allergic to mercury before receiving a mercury filling? I have not heard of any dentist testing for mercury allergy before placing dental amalgam. I know that I had never done it.

That statistic is the amount of people who may have an allergy to the metal itself. This does not include the larger number of people who have mercury vaporizing from their fillings over time and chronically suffer from its toxic effects. These people have an inability to excrete mercury, a genetic predisposition to sensitivity, have other toxins that are combining synergistically with mercury, or have already-challenged immune systems that cannot carry the toxic burden. In my experience, that is a much bigger number.

There are many other reasons that dentists are uniquely ignorant about the effects of mercury fillings on human health. Let's continue.

But if Mercury fillings are toxic, the ADA would tell me – wouldn't they?

After speaking with dentists about the "mercury issue," they most often comment that they thought the ADA had their best interests at heart and that if amalgam fillings were harmful, they would surely say so. Perhaps if you are a dentist reading this, you are about to find out that Santa Claus isn't real.

What would happen if the ADA came out tomorrow and said, "Oh, never mind what we said in the past. Those mercury fillings actually are toxic and unsafe for the public and dental staff." That would be the start of a litigation nightmare – lawsuits from dentists, dental staff, consumers, governmental agencies, and others. It could be the demise of the ADA and possibly bankrupt the dental manufacturers.

The ADA, born out of the mercury filling issue, took a position in the mid-1800s and has not changed its mind – even in the face of overwhelming scientific findings that link mercury fillings to the effects of toxic exposure and chronic disease. If you read the dental literature of those times, whenever someone brought up accounts of illness from the mercury fillings or studies, they would just quickly dismiss the ideas. It's like they just do not want to hear it. The ADA has dismissed any contradictions to their position since then.

If the ADA were an organization that supports scientific evidence, wouldn't they also support independent research to test and study the mercury filling? Over the course of 150 years, the ADA has not bothered to even study the matter in a credible fashion. Research efforts have been directed to reduce variation in amalgam composition and placement techniques – not toxic effects. In the past several decades, when the ADA was requested by some of their own membership to produce their scientific research or safety trials, they could not give any information.

The current ADA position is:

> "Dental amalgam is considered a safe, affordable and durable material that has been used to restore the teeth of more than 100 million Americans. It contains a mixture of metals such as silver, copper and tin, in addition to mercury, which binds these components into a hard, stable and safe substance. Dental amalgam has been studied and reviewed extensively, and has established a record of safety and effectiveness."

The ADA did not admit mercury vapor is released from the dental amalgam until 1984, even though concerned dentists and scientists have discussed it since the mid-1800s.
Now they say that mercury vapor is released from the filling, but it's not enough to hurt anyone. If they have come to the realization that mercury vapor is being released, wouldn't that call for multiple comprehensive studies to research or confirm this position?

The ADA has close relationships with dental amalgam manufacturers and governmental agencies, strengthened through millions of dollars in lobbying. They were also granted two patents (#4,018,600 and #4,078,921) for dental amalgam in the 1970s, which have since expired. These patents were held through their charitable and educational arm, the ADA Foundation. It has been a conflict of interest for the ADA to make comments about the safety of amalgam.

Sit down and shut up

To silence dentists about the controversy and to protect its position, the ADA adopted a gag rule in its "code of ethics." The ADA's gag rule is one of the reasons that the mercury controversy stays within dentistry. Organizations of mercury-free dentists don't have the funding needed for lobbyists, public relations firms and Political Action Committees (PACs) to compete with the power of the ADA. Just because the ADA is richer and bigger doesn't make them right.

The gag rule, a pillar of the ADA's agenda, blocks consumers from learning that the main component of amalgam is mercury with its possible toxic effects on their health. This gag rule directs dentists to abandon their duty to patient health care. Dentists are kept from initiating communications with patients about the risks of mercury dental fillings. The dentist must remain silent or face disciplinary action. This gag rule has unfortunately been enforced by many ADA dentist-dominated state dental boards.

Due to the efforts of Charlie Brown from Consumers for Dental Choice going to every region around the country to challenge the gag rule in the courts, some dentists are free to discuss mercury-free dentistry. The California Dental Board repealed its gag rule in 1999. Many states (but not all) have now followed this legal standing. It is time for every state dental board to stop enforcing this gag rule and allow patients the right of informed consent.

According to the ADA Code of Professional Conduct, 5.A.1. - Dental Amalgam and Other Restorative Materials:

> "Based on current scientific data the ADA has determined that the removal of amalgam restorations from the non-allergic patient for the alleged purpose of removing toxic substances from the body, when such treatment is performed solely at the recommendation of the dentist, is improper and unethical. The same principle of veracity

applies to the dentist's recommendation concerning the removal of any dental restorative material."

In the 1980s, I had a radio show in Los Angeles called "Smile Your Way to Health." I even interviewed Dr. Hal Huggins and Dr. Joyal Taylor about the amalgam issue. Perhaps because of my affiliation with UCLA, or numerous celebrity patients, or because I hadn't been a member of the ADA since 1970, I was given a pass - or maybe no one was listening.

But I have known many dentists throughout this country who have been disciplined for speaking out against the use of amalgam. Many dentists are still extremely cautious in states that suppress the idea that amalgams may be harmful.

Recently, during the ongoing negotiations of the UNEP treaty, Californians for Green Dentistry, other concerned citizens and I were asked by Charlie Brown, also of the World Alliance for Mercury-Free Dentistry, to go to various city councils in California and ask them to adopt a resolution to support the global ban on mercury. We were successful in doing so in Malibu and Costa Mesa, CA, as well as a few other cities. We did this because showing that independent governmental bodies support taking action against mercury products would be helpful during negotiations.

Interestingly enough, just before the City of Malibu took a vote, Mayor John Sibert – a retired chemical engineer, told the City Council about his experience with the Planning Commission and a construction project. He said soil tests for the construction site showed high levels of mercury, which would not have been expected for the area. He went on to say that upon further investigation, they found that a dental office had previously occupied the location. He was fully aware of the potential for pollution and human poisoning from mercury dental products. The resolution passed unanimously.

While we were going to various cities to ask them to adopt the resolutions, sometimes we were met with opposition from the local dental societies. In fact, the California Dental Association sent out a letter to the regional leaders to watch their local city council agendas for amalgam-related items on the calendar. I saw a copy of that letter.

I was also told by other people organizing the City Council appearances that some dental association members were threatened by the local dental societies that if they were to participate with us, they would be expelled from the organization or lose some of the benefits afforded by the ADA, like insurance. We had several dentists cancel their appearances at the last minute because of these threats.

Information lockup at the California Dental Board

In 2002, a mercury-free dentist and colleague of mine, Chet Yokoyama, DDS, was appointed to a seat on the California Dental Board and served as Chairman of the Dental Materials Fact Sheet Committee. By law, California was required to create a fact sheet to be given to people when they are exposed to a chemical known to cause birth defects and reproductive harm, which would include dental amalgam. He testified before the Subcommittee on Human Rights and Wellness at a US Congressional Hearing, regarding California's Compliance with Dental Amalgam Disclosure Policies.

I feel his testimony describing the actions of members of the California Dental Board was so concerning, that a summation would lose the flavor of injustice done upon the residents of California. I have inserted it here, in its entirety. This is Dr. Yokoyama's opening statement to the Committee on January 26, 2004:

> "Chairman Burton and Ranking Member Diane Watson, thank you very much for giving me the opportunity to speak here today.
>
> I am speaking today as an individual dentist. I am a member of the Dental Board of California. I do not speak for the dental board and I am giving my opinions only.
>
> So I come today to tell you about an extremely disappointing turn of events. This turn of events directly applies to the subject of California's compliance with the dental amalgam disclosure policies. As you are well aware, the California law required the dental board to produce a fact sheet on the risks and efficacies of filling materials. A second law mandated that these facts be given to every patient. And this would, of course, disclose the health risks of mercury in dental amalgam to the public. And to this end I have given my time and my energy.

I have been proud to serve as the chairman of the Dental Materials Fact Sheet Committee. And when I approached the existing document, I quickly realized that it contained several statements that seemed to be incorrect. I called for a hearing on the scientific evidence of health risk from mercury in the amalgam. We learned that there are scientists with relevant scientific studies and publishing in relevant scientific journals. When I found there was evidence of a substantial health risk to members of our California population, I felt it was my duty to give a clear warning concerning that risk.

It is a risk of exposure to a chemical known to the State of California to cause birth defects and reproductive harm. A risk that is a fact in California law known as Proposition 65.

As chairman of the Dental Materials Fact Sheet Committee, I was able to develop a document that included this warning. I developed this document over a period of time. There were many meetings, emails, phone calls and discussions. There was stakeholder input. Dentists gave their opinions. There was public debate. The dental board had a hearing and in public view discussed the contents of the draft fact sheet multiple times. I dotted all my I's and crossed all my T's. This process was done by the book, step-by-step.

So why am I so extremely disappointed? I shall explain further.

Last year at the July board meeting this draft document was brought to the board and it was voted 7 to 1 to approve the idea of including the warning I spoke of and a message to pregnant women and parents. The board then requested that the Department of Consumer Affairs make this document into a brochure and make sure that the language was consumer-friendly. It was agreed upon by the board that at the next meeting in November 2003 the board would take the final vote.

Well just before the meeting in November the California Dental Association sent out a letter to each board member saying that the Prop 65 warning, the warning about the exposure to mercury and its connection with birth defects and reproductive harm, was false and misleading. And it must be said here that it was the same CDA that sent out the same warning to dentists. That warning stated ``Dental Amalgam... exposes you to mercury, a substance known to the State of California to cause birth defects and reproductive harm.'' The letter sent to the board members had an opinion from their expert that this statement was false and misleading. A very odd chain of events, not easily explained. Nevertheless, this is a matter for the Cal-EPA scientists to be notified of, because this warning is a matter of law in the State of California.

So even with this strange letter, the dental board had its meeting in November and after deliberations, again voted to approve the brochure, 8 to zero. The board agreed that it was the right format and ``95 percent complete.'' The committee was asked to make minor changes and bring it back in one month for a final vote. That vote was to occur by the end of the year 2003. So I quickly did the board requested editing and sent the changes off to the other member of the committee for her approval.

The other committee member was initially too busy. I waited an appropriate period of time and re-requested her answer. To my surprise, she sent me a completely new draft fact sheet. This was laid out professionally and was complete, in brochure form already. Several questions were in my mind. Where did this new version come from? Why did the president not ask for an explanation? Why did the president not direct us to work from the twice-approved document that was clearly what the board expected? Then there was no meeting in December.

I was upset by these developments. And then came the most disturbing turn of events. At the beginning of the year, I was sent an email that said that I was no longer the chairman of the committee, and that there was an entirely new committee and a new agenda. My attempts to comply with the California Dental Amalgam Disclosure Policies had been side tracked.

I hope that you will urge the dental board to push forward for full disclosure.

And I'd like to mention just a couple of things while I was working on this committee that I found. I found several facts that make it even more important that the dental board continue on its quest to bring full disclosure of health risks in order to protect the people of California.

First, to depend on the FDA as the source of safety of dental amalgam is invalid. These are things I learned along the way in my opinion. It is often assumed that the FDA has studied this health risk carefully. For that matter, it is often said that the FDA has approved dental amalgam as safe. I found quite the contrary. The FDA claims no jurisdiction over mixed dental amalgam because it is mixed by the dentist. The dentist is the manufacturer, mixing the mercury and silver particles in the office and thereby manufacturing the final mixed product that goes into the teeth. The FDA therefore has made no classification, does not regulate, has not studied and does not approve the mixed amalgam.

The FDA also did not study or demand studies to classify the separate ingredients, which they have classified the separate mercury and the separate silver fillings. The separate ingredients were simply ``grandfathered'' in.

As late as January 15, 2004, the head of the Dental Devices Division of the FDA has said that ``the agency did propose to classify'' in other words approve, and I'm putting that word in there to help you out. ``The agency did propose to classify the encapsulated form of amalgam approximately 1 year ago and at the present time that process is on hold.'' When asked why, she said, ``The status of the classification as being on hold is awaiting additional information from a third review of the literature on dental amalgam that is being conducted.'' So even the encapsulated form, which would be the closest to the actual substance that dentists use to fill teeth is not classified, and therefore not approved.

So the second realization was that the ADA/CDA, the ADA and by extension the CDA, has argued successfully in California courts that ``The ADA owes no legal duty of care to protect the public from allegedly dangerous products used by dentists. The ADA did not manufacture, design, supply or install the mercury-containing amalgams. The ADA does not control those who do. The ADA's only alleged involvement in the product was to provide information regarding its use. Dissemination of information relating to the practice of dentistry does not create a duty of care to protect the public from potential injury.''

So this puts the burden squarely on the shoulders of the individual dentist who is "manufacturing" the amalgam and therefore responsible.

So I found three important questions: One, has the FDA approved dental amalgam for safety? My opinion is no.

Two, does the ADA/CDA owe a duty of care to protect the patient from health risks from dental amalgam? In my opinion no.

Three, does the dental board have the responsibility to protect the public from known sources of health risk? Yes.

Then it logically follows that:

One, amalgam is 50 percent mercury? Yes.

Two, mercury vapor constantly is emitted and goes to the organs of the body? Yes.

Three, amalgam is the predominant source of mercury exposure in people who have amalgam filling? Yes.

Four, dental amalgam exposes you to mercury, a substance known to the State of California to cause birth defects and reproductive harm. Yes.

Therefore, dental amalgam is unsuitable for use in pregnant women and pregnant women should be clearly warned.

I shall continue to press for full disclosure of the risks of dental amalgam to patients in order to better enable them to make informed choices.

And I would just like to say that I am disappointed with the absence of the California Dental Association. We are trying to come to an agreement, but it is difficult if you do not come to the table. And I am disappointed with the absence of any of the board members or representatives of the board, I will just say that. And I thank you for your time."

This is a perfect example of how the California Dental Association, which is under the self-appointed authority of the ADA, consistently hides information from dentists and the public. They are able to squash any attempts at informed consent at every turn.

And apparently the brochure was effective in convincing the general public that mercury fillings are safe.

A word about that brochure . . .

During the course of writing this book, I had shown a significant portion of the manuscript to a friend who isn't involved in dentistry, except for the fact that they do have teeth. While saying that they thought the book was good, they sent to me, without comment, a brochure from the Dental Board of California entitled, "The Facts About Fillings." Interestingly enough, this is the exact brochure that is thoroughly discussed in the previous testimony.

In an email, I thanked my friend for giving me the brochure and pointed out that this was the same brochure of interest in Chapter 8, and is now eleven years old. I also mentioned that since then, the World Health Organization referenced in the brochure, has taken the position of supporting the global phase down of dental mercury, and that just only last month, the country of Brazil went mercury free!

But this action by my friend brings up a poignant observation, and it really made me aware of something that I had not previously considered. Within the general public, there are a lot of people that believe statements made by governmental agencies, without discernment. They trust that the FDA, their dental board, and that even the ADA really has their best interest at heart. If the Dental Board of California says that mercury emitting from a tooth doesn't pose a risk, then it must be okay.

How do we convince the masses that think money, legal recourse, and political influence aren't a major factor in positions taken by a governmental agency for a wide array of health, safety, and product issues? I think that is a topic for another book.

But the ADA surely wouldn't mislead the public

Consumers mistakenly buy into the notion that the ADA has concern for their safety. The ADA is a trade association, and by their own admission, feels no duty to the public or to protect the consumer. In a 1995 lawsuit about amalgam (*W.H. Tolhurst vs. Johnson and Johnson Consumer Products, Inc.; Engelhard Corporation; ABE Dental, Inc.; the American Dental Association, et al.,*) the ADA legal brief stated: "The ADA owes no legal duty of care to protect the public from allegedly dangerous products used by dentists."

Clearly, they are not interested in protecting the public against toxic effects of amalgam fillings. They said so themselves. Their position was that the dentist mixed the amalgam and he is on his own for any liability of damages. The ADA went further on to say:

"The ADA did not manufacture, design, supply or install the mercury-containing amalgams. The ADA does not control those who do. The ADA's only alleged involvement in the product was to provide information regarding its use. Dissemination of information relating to the practice of dentistry does not create a duty of care to protect the public from potential injury."

The ADA will vehemently fight for the use of dental amalgam, but they won't take responsibility for what they say to the dental profession or the public.

Jim Love, an attorney who was involved with the *Tolhurst vs. Johnson and Johnson Consumer Products, Inc., et al* case, recently discussed the stronghold that the ADA has on blocking information from dentists and consumers. He stated:

"... In fact, the ADA is the profession of dentistry. They set the standard of care: they set the standards for accreditation of dental schools; they set the standards that are adhered to by dental boards. In fact, the dental board members are almost invariably staffed by members of the ADA. The ADA staffs the dental division of the FDA. They so pervasively control everything that happens in the regulatory context throughout this country that they are firmly in control of all of the decisions that pertain to the profession. So for the ADA to say that they are just out promoting the interests of the profession of dentistry is a fraud on the American public. It's not true at all."

Blocking information about dental mercury is a widespread and concerted effort – and not all that difficult for them to accomplish.

What about the FDA? They would ban the dental amalgam if it were bad; right?

Let's start with the FDA's current position on the mercury filling. Well, they have basically vomited out the same position as the ADA, without ever requiring manufacturers of amalgams to perform any safety studies on this product – a product that contains a known neurotoxin, mercury.

When the FDA regulatory authority was extended to medical devices in 1976, the FDA pronounced acceptance of amalgam fillings and "grandfathered" their approval under the Generally

Recognized as Safe (GRAS) category, due to its long term usage, even before the existence of the FDA.

To define the level of risk, devices are given classifications.

Class I: lowest risk devices and requires only general safety controls.

Class II: moderate risk devices and requires special controls.

Class III: highest risk devices and requires manufactures to provide extensive proof of safety and formal FDA premarket approval.

In 1987, the alloy and mercury were classified separately since at that time, they were normally sold separately and then mixed by the dentist. Mercury was classified as Class I and dental alloy as Class II. What? Dental Mercury was put in the same category as Q-Tips and Band-Aids?

For many years, the FDA avoided properly classifying dental amalgam as it began to be sold in a capsulated form. Dental amalgam had not been classified until after the FDA was petitioned by consumer groups in 1991. This was the same year that the World Health Organization reported that exposure to dental mercury is higher than fish, seafood, water and air – and the same year that Sweden announced a plan to ban amalgam fillings.

In 1994, the Dental Products Panel recommended that the FDA classify amalgam as a Class II device. In 1997, after a review of the body of literature through 1997, they found no support for claims of adverse health effects from amalgam, except for rare allergic or hypersensitive reactions. In 2004, a similar review was done resulting in a similar finding. No clinical studies were ever done.

From 2006 to 2009, there were many interactions between the FDA and consumer groups and mercury-free dentistry organizations, including several hearings at which consumers and dental staff testified about their injuries or dentists about their experiences with the toxicity of dental amalgam. It came down to the FDA classifying the dental amalgam capsule as a Class II medical device, which really has very little impact on clinical dentistry. Warnings required by manufacturers to dentists, but not by dentists to patients.

The proper classification for mercury fillings should be Class III, which would require a manufacturer to prove safety. Keeping the dental amalgam in Class II avoids safety testing. This is something that is implanted in a child's head, two inches from his brain and may be there for a decade or two. As a country, we cannot be bothered to test it?

Manufacturers, in close relationships with the ADA, will not test for safety. They are unwilling to spend millions of dollars to prove that mercury is safe. We all know mercury is not safe. If the dental amalgam is ever determined to be a Class III device, it is likely the manufacturers would just let the time elapse for safety trials, and then pull the product off of the market. Declaring the dental amalgam a Class III device would basically mean the eventual ban of the product, since it would not be available.

The bonds between the ADA, the FDA and dental amalgam manufacturers are very real and very strong. FDA Commissioner Martha Hamburg presided over the FDA's long-delayed classification of dental amalgam. She still had stock options from her board seat at Henry Schein, one of the largest amalgam manufacturers, up until her recusal, which she did quietly only after being put under pressure to do so. The fix was in, and Henry Schein thanked her for her service.

The power of the dental industry and its anti-regulatory lobby adds up to an apparent unwillingness to put public health above all else.

A lot of dentists say there is no problem with the Mercury filling

I have also had many discussions with dentists who argue strongly in favor of the mercury filling. It's difficult to know why a dentist is so resistant to the notion that mercury is still toxic, even in the form of the dental filling, but I do have some ideas. After all, I was one of them. These are good people, and most all of them have good intentions.

1. **Some dentists really don't believe that the ADA would mislead them or that their training was faulty.** They paid a lot for that degree, and it would be difficult to think that such a significant part of their work is based on something that is not true.

2. **For some dentists, realizing that they have been putting a toxic substance in thousands of people over the years is just too much to bear.** I have my own guilty feelings about what I did in my father's mouth, my children's mouths, and teaching all those dentists to perpetuate the systematic poisoning of men, women and children.

3. **Some dentists actually don't care.** There are some people who went into dentistry because of the money, and if everyone else is placing mercury fillings, then they have a right to make a profit. These are the dentists who look at patients as conversions into cash. I am sorry to say that I have met too many of these dentists.

4. **Some dentists are not aware of any ill effects of having placed a mercury filling.** For example, if a patient experiences neurological symptoms like tingling or dizziness, they aren't likely to relate it to something done by the dentist – but perhaps they should. As we will discuss in a subsequent chapter, mercury toxicity is very difficult to diagnose, and symptoms often don't present in the mouth.

5. **Some dentists think that we need a cheaper alternative for people who are financially disadvantaged.** Well, lead paint is cheaper, too. Poisoning poor people is not a good policy.

In 2011, I gave a course in Los Angeles about mercury-safe dentistry. We advertised to the general population of mainstream dentists. The ads each contained a different theme, such as protecting the environment, healthy dentistry, and physical symptoms of toxicity. I asked the attendees what influenced them to come to the class. The dentists who came responded primarily to an advertisement about the symptoms of mercury toxicity, and how they may be sick from mercury exposure. Therefore, it was their own symptoms and health that motivated the dentists to learn more about the dental amalgam. Some of them spoke about how they were experiencing symptoms like lethargy, tremors, irritability, and memory loss, but couldn't get a diagnosis from allopathic medicine. They expressed relief that they now know that they may be mercury toxic, know how to properly test for it, and can do something about it.

Tantrums, finger shaking, insults ... on both sides

After a dentist or consumer becomes aware that the dental profession has perpetuated the idea that amalgam is safe for more than 150 years, they often get angry. Sometimes they get really angry. I have seen some pretty poor behavior on the part of my colleagues during public exchanges with people on the pro-amalgam side of the debate. It then becomes a loud, crass argument involving both sides. You can see it in the comments section of any website with an article about dental amalgams. It can get just plain nasty.

I have been embarrassed by the behavior of some anti-amalgam dentists and consumers. In fact, in the 1980s, when I had a prominent anti-mercury dentist on my radio show, a woman representing the California Dental Association called into the show, who was clearly pro-amalgam. My guest proceeded to insult her in a very personal manner, attributing her inability to comprehend the anti-amalgam position to her menstrual cycle. This anti-mercury dentist made numerous and invaluable contributions to mercury-free dentistry, but his often rude vocalizations affected the progress of the anti-mercury movement. He was angry about the injustice, but offending the woman in such a manner likely turned off people who might have otherwise opened their mind.

When you attend public debates about mercury fillings, they often include finger shaking and contempt. I don't believe this type of behavior will expedite the abolishment of dental mercury. I think we need to remember that these are people, most of which don't have malicious intentions. They are only repeating what they have been told, and sometimes feel threatened by change. Yes, there are some people with enough power to make changes that expressly perpetuate the myth of amalgam safety, but we usually don't see those people. They are the ones who send the foot soldiers out for the pro-amalgam cause.

But also keep in mind, the anti-amalgam dentist is often someone who has been extremely ill from mercury toxicity or have a family member that has been a victim of an unsafe mercury removal or placement of a neurotoxin that they didn't know was in the dental filling.

Poor behavior by the mercury-free community hurts the cause more than it helps. We need to remember to practice compassion, act professionally, and represent the mercury-poisoned victims in a respectable manner. I understand the anger, but we need to become the observer and come from a kind-hearted and empathetic place.

It is not to say that people on the pro-amalgam side don't misbehave. I have consistently seen extremely rude and condescending behavior there, too. We need to keep in mind that oftentimes, these people may also be mercury toxic and are an unwitting victim. It's just that it is most important that the people who are working to get mercury out of dentistry do it with dignity and grace.

By the way, did you ever notice you don't see pro-amalgam consumer activists? The only people really passionate about keeping a neurotoxin in dentistry are dentists ... oh, and the ADA ... and the manufacturers.

Is there a way out for the ADA?

I would like to welcome the ADA to the evolving profession of dentistry. The ADA has an opportunity to move forward, mercury free. They know they can do it. It would be smarter for them to not wait until they are forced. If the ADA waits until there is so much public and professional anger and mistrust against them, they may not survive or may slip into irrelevancy.

They could take a position that upon further investigation with new studies and information, they have decided to remove dental amalgam from availability in dentistry, and will make a sincere effort to educate dentists about safe mercury removal. Over the past 200 years, dentistry has taken enormous strides in oral care and other dental procedures. It is perfectly acceptable to evolve into a dental profession that considers the impact of dental choices on the whole body, truthfully informs the patient of risks and benefits, and learns from its mistakes.

Taking mercury out of dentistry and removing existing amalgam fillings safely is the most important thing. That alone would be worth not placing blame and acting punitively.

Let's give them a pass. I would, wouldn't you?

And maybe we can get them to drop fluoride, while we're at it.

Chapter 9

The Mouth is a Mirror of the Body

This evolution in dentistry goes far beyond eliminating the use of mercury fillings. Biological dentistry has a true appreciation of the science of the human body and the relationship of the mouth to the rest of the body. Biological dentistry is not a branch of dentistry. It is an awareness integrated in the process of restoring the patient's mouth to optimal health, with the acknowledgment of the impact that process has on the rest of the body. Today, only 1% of dentists study this concept and make it a part of their practice.

I am in awe at the amount of information the mouth and its related environment can tell us. What happens in the body is often reflected in the mouth. The Father of Modern Medicine, Sir William Osler said in the 1800s, "The mouth is the mirror of the body which reflects systemic diseases."

I want to share with you some extraordinary observations I have made in my 50 years in dentistry. I believe these experiences made me a better dentist and played a significant role in my evolution as a human being.

When we, as dentists, are mindful of the various elements of the human experience, acutely aware of the sacred responsibility we hold when we treat the mouth of another person – and we are humbled by the sensitivity, complexity, and beauty of the design of the human body and spirit – it is in that moment we do our best work, in service to the well-being of the patient, and we are grateful for the fulfilling experience of restoring health to that person.

The mouth is a sacred part of the body. It is a highly sensitive entrance to the body. It is where we verbalize our thoughts, where we eat our food, where we kiss and experience intimacy, and where we laugh and sing. We instinctually cover our mouth when we are afraid or surprised. We may bite to defend ourselves. We look at other people's mouths and make judgments based on its size, color, condition and reflection of the current state of emotion. We socialize with our mouths, even from great distances. Some of us will use our mouth to chant the word "Om" to tune into the vibration of the universe. It is considered the frequency of energy that connects and joins all things together.

There is also neurological sensitivity of the mouth that is well demonstrated by the fact that 5 of the 12 cranial nerves that exit from the brain through openings in the skull, have functions associated with the mouth. Some are motor nerves, which send impulses from the brain that tell muscles to move. These are also sensory nerves, which allow the brain to detect sensation in and around the mouth. Other nerves have special functions such as detecting taste or regulating the salivary glands.

We all have an innate sensitivity of the mouth, for which I have grown to deeply respect. Some people have a fear of dentists because of a previous traumatic experience. There is a high correlation between women who were orally sexually abused and dental phobia, which is all the more reason to approach patients with great care and respect for this most sensitive part of the body. Throughout my dental career, I always asked the patient permission to enter their mouth before starting any dental procedure. For some, being in the dental chair is disturbing, so we must respect the possibility of previous trauma.

The mouth is a most fascinating part of the body. It can tell you things without saying a word.

Memory and crystals

Teeth are a remarkable part of the body. In simple terms, teeth are enamel covering bone. Bone is closely related to dentin, which is the foundation for the tooth. Dentin is covered by enamel, which is the hardest substance in the body. I think of teeth as crystals. Microscopically, dentin and enamel are a crystalline material.

Now, think about this: Is it possible that your teeth as "crystals" store memory? Crystals are able to store a lot of information. Small computer chips store millions of pieces of data. The enamel in teeth is made up of millions of tiny crystals. Is it possible that each one is like a computer chip and can hold a lifetime of information? The brain is a bio-computer. Could the teeth record memories or information? Interestingly enough, studies have shown that people that have lost their teeth, especially molars, have a decline in memory.

Is there a connection? Maybe someday science will study the crystalline properties of teeth to see if they store information. Just because it has not been studied, doesn't mean that we should just dismiss it. I believe in respecting the possibility, as I have seen the human body reveal some remarkable and seemingly impossible things.

Energy pathways

When we study the body in the Eastern viewpoint, the cells in the body are vibrating. There are twelve cell salts vibrating in 90% water. That vibration – that chi – that yin-yang – that Holy Spirit – that bio-plasma – that electromagnetic force – is what holds things together.

It forms pathways in the body, referred to as meridians. Electronically, the bio-physicist can see that there is a way to record that flow of energy and to determine the absence of flow or blockages. Optimal health is when everything is flowing freely. But because of free will, we can block that flow or that flow can be blocked traumatically or toxically. Therefore, clearing those energetic pathways is the road back to health. This is a widely known universal principle outside of the United States.

In this country, we battle disease by treating the symptoms of the disease process. When you have a pain, you can numb it with a pain pill. When you have an infection, you can treat the inflammation and bacteria, which result from a breakdown in the immune system. The bacteria will only show up when the host is susceptible. This allopathic, mainstream medicine rarely looks at why the person is susceptible in the first place.

The principles of acupuncture apply to the mouth. The teeth are connected to the body's electrical system. Now, let's add the crystalline properties of the teeth to the electronic circuitry. How would the teeth not be connected to this energetic system? Mainstream dentistry ignores this connection.

Two doctors from Germany, Fritz Kramer, DDS and Reinhold Voll, MD, of the International Society for Electro-Acupuncture, identified that a particular organ or part of the body is energetically or electrically connected to each tooth. Their work was later confirmed by a physician-dentist, Dr. Gleditsch, and again by Thomas Rau, MD, who also found that similar relationships and body maps exist in the mouth.

Each tooth is related to an acupuncture meridian that is connected to an organ meridian, muscle, vertebrae, spinal cord, cranial nerve, and endocrine gland. Whenever a tooth is irritated, stimulated, or traumatized from a toxic dental material and an electromagnetic current, its associated body part may also be involved. At first the associated area may become irritated and inflamed, which may lead to an acute symptom of physiological distress. If left untreated, eventually, the associated organ, muscle, or nerve may become degenerative and diseased.

When we look at the meridian tooth charts compiled by Drs. Voll and Kramer, we see that the teeth can communicate energetically to various parts of the body. For example, the molars are associated with the stomach; the canines or eye teeth go to the liver and the eyes. In the resource section of this book, there is a link to where you can use an interactive meridian tooth chart to consider the condition of your own mouth.

Hold those thoughts about the body's electrical system for a moment, because we need to talk about some conditions in the mouth and teeth that will influence health in the rest of the body because of electronics.

Galvanic reactions – the battery in the mouth

A battery is created when two dissimilar metals are connected by way of a substance that contains ions, called an electrolyte. Dissimilar metals means that each metal has a different atomic structure, leading to a positive or negative polarity in the flow of ions. Any pair of positively and negatively charged metals separated by a conductor will behave as a battery. This interaction of metals to create an electrical charge is called galvanism.

We are not born with galvanic reactions in our mouth. The incompatible materials in dentistry create these reactions. When two dissimilar metals are placed in the mouth - with saliva being the electrolyte - then a battery is created, meaning a galvanic reaction takes place. This is the production and flow of ions, and is a principle in electronics – and it happens in the mouth.

An effect of galvanism occurs when a mercury filling (also containing zinc, tin, and copper) exists in the mouth with a gold crown or filling. These dissimilar metals in conjunction with saliva constitute an electric cell. Pain or inflammation may be experienced when the dissimilar metals interact, the circuit is created, and a flow of electrical current passes through the pulp. The current flows from metal to metal through the dentine and tissue fluids of both teeth resulting in discomfort and tooth sensitivity. Even once the pain subsides, galvanization continues to disturb the body balance.

Mercury readily forms alloys with other metals. It is used to extract gold during the mining process where the mercury amalgamates with gold. These two metals have an excellent binding relationship. Remember my sock drawer where I kept that vial of mercury? At times, the lid would loosen and there were small amoeba-like droplets of mercury rolling around the drawer. I previously mentioned that as a boy, I received a gold-plated watch as a gift for my Catholic Confirmation and kept it in the sock drawer. The watch was ruined by the mercury in the drawer and turned gray. The mercury amalgamated with the gold watch.

One of the effects of galvanism is the "mercury tattoo." On a tooth with a mercury filling, sometimes you can see the gum tissue has also turned gray or black. Most dentists are not aware of the main source of mercury tattoos. Because of galvanism and the electric currents caused by mixed metals in the mouth, the amalgam accumulates in the tissue near the teeth with large fillings or metal crowns over amalgam. Certain periodontal bacteria produce hydrogen sulfide, a toxic gas. This combines with elemental mercury to produce mercuric sulfide, a black solid which precipitates on the gum or cheek. Amalgam tattoos are not a sign the dentist was sloppy with amalgam placement or removal, but that bacteria have produced hydrogen sulfide and that there was mercury present to combine with it. The mercury and other metals will move to other parts of the body in significant amounts over time.

Those of us who have practiced dentistry over the years, have seen time and time again, decay occurring around crowns and fillings. When I became aware of these electrical principles taking place, I began to see decay that would occur between the two teeth with the fillings. Was the decay accelerated due to electrical currents along with bacteria in those areas? Acids produced by galvanic reactions may be present even in a very clean mouth.

Back to the meridians

Earlier, I briefly went through the energy pathways in the body, which ideally should be open and unblocked. The electrical currents created by the metals used in fillings and root canals can conflict both with each other and with the body's electrical system, leading to interferences and disturbances in the body's own bioelectrical currents.

The quickest growing tissues in the body are the mucosal tissues of the mouth. They rejuvenate every 48 hours. It is an early-warning system of conditions occurring in the rest of the body. When there is a change in circulation in an environment, the vibrational areas of one part of the body can affect a certain tooth through this energy pathway system.

We can then ask the question, why does one tooth decay more than other teeth? Is there a change of circulation or stimulation on that meridian that causes an interruption or acceleration in the demineralization process? Or is the decay process caused by acidophilic (acid-loving) bacteria? Are certain bacteria more present in certain areas of the body? Is there a circulatory disturbance in another part of the body that is affecting a particular tooth?

There is an electrical connection, a meridian connection, and a cause-and-effect system taking place. What's causing the tooth to decay? Is that the body part that has changed frequency or is the tooth causing the body part to malfunction?

What does a dentist do with this information? Once I understood the relationship of the teeth to the rest of the body, and with much observation and discernment, I have been able to alert patients to possible correlations to other conditions occurring in their body. Over the years, while diagnosing the condition of a patient's teeth, I have been able to consistently see those correlations.

For instance, if I saw a gold crown on Tooth #14 and a mercury filling on Tooth #15, which happens to involve the stomach meridian, I would be suspicious that this patient may have digestive problems. And more often than not, in reviewing the patient's health history, they had noted a digestive disorder. When you see this phenomenon over and over again – well, it's no longer a surprise. Should a person with a stomachache go to a dentist?

Perhaps they should include a biological dentist in their program for improving their heath.

The American Dental Association has a similar position on galvanism as it does on mercury fillings. Even though considerable amounts of scientific literature references the problems caused by galvanic reactions in the mouth, the dental profession establishment hopes these findings go unnoticed and discourages dentists from speaking of it. Because of this, there is only a relatively small number of dentists that have an understanding of biological dentistry, and it is the patient that is left uninformed.

The Tooth: Wanted dead or alive – root canal controversy

The biting question in dentistry - even among biological dentists – is do we always remove a tooth once it has died? As humans, we are the only species that are willing to keep a dead body part. Once the nerve is removed from the tooth, it is dead. The only thing that tooth can do now is gather bacteria, regardless of how skilled the dentist believes he is at sterilizing the canals of the root. In dental school, we are taught to save the tooth at all costs. Well, it does cost a lot to keep a dead tooth, and I am not talking about money.

As mentioned before, the live, healthy tooth is made up of dentin, which is very hard and consists of a large number of dentinal tubules. These tiny tubes allow fluid to come from the central root canal through the dentin, and out through the outer layer of the root, to the bone and gum tissue outside of the tooth. This comprises a circulatory system designed to nourish and maintain the hydrostatic pressure of the root canal, the nerves and blood vessels in the canal, and the gum and bone tissue surrounding the tooth. This fluid flows from the tubules of the tooth and is picked up by the lymphatic system to go through detoxification channels.

During a root canal procedure, the dentist tries to remove the nerves, blood vessels and clean out the dead tissue. The canal is sterilized and filled with a sterile material. This process usually alleviates pain and leaves the tooth intact, making it serviceable.

However, when the canal is filled, the fluid is removed, and the tooth becomes dehydrated. The circulatory system of the tubules becomes stagnant. Anaerobic bacteria, which do not require oxygen to live, digest the dead tissue and flourish in the tubules. This bacteria spreads through your body from the blood supply and lymphatics that surround the dead tooth. This toxic effect will go to all the organ systems and can lead to various degenerative conditions, such as musculoskeletal disorders, autoimmune diseases, digestive issues, cancer, depression, and more.

People tend to want to keep the tooth, even if it is dead. It is important to always discuss the potential consequences of this decision. I would let them know that this tooth would now always be a burden on their body and to stay vigilant regarding the area of the body that the tooth is associated with, according to the tooth meridians. For example, if the root canal was going to be performed on the front tooth, #8, then I told them to watch for health changes in their urinary or genital areas.

I also advised them to make sure they were proactively keeping their immune system as strong as possible. When the immune system is weakened, the toxic effects of a root canal may take hold of their overall health. I would also tell them that if in the future, they develop a systemic disorder, they should let their physician know that they have a dead tooth in their mouth. This will assist the physician in diagnosis and possible treatment for the condition.

I did not perform root canals in my dental practice. If a patient insisted on keeping the tooth after telling them about my concerns for keeping the tooth, I would refer them to an endodontist who agrees with our attempt to use biocompatible materials. I do not recommend root canals for anyone. However, each person has a right to make their own decision.

For myself, I have never had a root canal. When one of my teeth developed an abscess and became painful, I had it extracted and gave that tooth a proper burial.

Implants - titanium and ceramic, or not at all

Implants have become very popular in the United States. I hear commercials on television claiming to reconstruct people's mouth in just one day. Having implants placed in the jaw is a very big decision, and the mainstream dental profession has not fully explored the long-term implications of implant dentistry. It is troublesome to me that dentists take the implant process so lightly. In looking at websites for implant dentists, there is rarely a mention of possible side effects, which include bacteria buildup, infection, inflammation, rejection, trapped nerves, allergies or interaction with other dentistry.

As I have always said, anything other than a healthy tooth is a compromise. Once an additional burden is placed on the body, it will depend on the susceptibility of the host and whether or not the body can handle the burden.

Like the mercury filling, titanium or metal implants can create oral galvanism in the mouth. When a metal implant is placed, there are three parts to the device: the implant, the abutment and the restoration – usually a crown. This means placing even more different metal types in the mouth. The implant is titanium, the abutment is a metal connector to the crown that may be made of titanium, surgical stainless steel or gold, and then the crown may contain metal materials itself.

Metal implants, including titanium, become corroded. The electrical currents in the mouth increase the rate at which the ions that are released react with the organs of the body. This may lead to increased sensitivity, opportunity for inflammation, neurological disturbances, and potential autoimmune disorders. The increased rate of corrosion increases the chance of developing toxic reactions to metals. Even fluoride toothpaste can corrode metal implants.

Titanium is not considered to be a biocompatible material for the mouth. Cases of intolerance to these metal implants are on the rise due to an increase in people receiving them. A recent study followed 56 patients who developed severe health problems after receiving titanium-based dental implants. The patients described medical problems including nerve, muscle and joint pain, neurological problems, chronic fatigue syndrome, depression, as well as inflammation and skin rashes.

When a patient cannot tolerate the titanium implant, one option is to have the metal implant removed or perhaps replaced with a more biocompatible material such as a ceramic implant. The ceramic implant manufacturers claim patients who have had metal implants replaced have reported reduced metal sensitivity overall and long-term health improvement in many cases.

The development of ceramic dental implants shows them to be more biocompatible to the human body, due to their poor electrical conductivity. These non-metal implants do not create a galvanic effect when compared to metal implants. Studies have shown that osseo-integration (the way an implant is integrated into the surrounding bone) is very similar to titanium. Ceramic implants also have a comparable rate of performance and durability.

In my dental practice, we often performed restorative work on celebrities, who were reluctant to use any type of removable device like a denture or partial denture. So they were inclined to choose the implant option to restore their mouth to a "television smile" appearance. For much of my career, there was no other option for an implant than metal. The ceramic implants came at the end of my chairside career, and even then, I didn't feel they were ready for use. Since then, ceramic implants have been developed into a more viable non-metal option.

There is more to consider than metal vs. non-metal implants. The fact is that the extracted tooth and its surrounding area have been compromised by infection. Normally, when a tooth is extracted, the body fills in the missing tooth area of the bone. However, if the membrane of the tooth or residual infection is left behind and the area cannot completely heal or fill in, a cavitation may result. It seems the bone cells on either side sense the existence of the periodontal membrane and respond as if the tooth is still there. This appears to be one common cause of cavitations. It leaves a hole or spongy area in the jaw and can be painful and harbor bacteria.

If an implant is placed into the bone where the previous tooth had a root canal procedure, and the bone was insufficiently cleaned out when the tooth was extracted, then the bone may still be infected and the implant is being placed into a chronically infected bone. There is no reason to believe that bacteria won't continue to inhabit the areas around the implant and then multiply and attract more bacteria. When anything is implanted into bone, it will create an autoimmune challenge. This situation creates an attraction for microorganisms.

Further, Dr. Hal Huggins did considerable research concerning dental implants and bone grafts – which are often used in the implant process – and through DNA analysis found large and various amounts of strains of microorganisms that would be concerning to anyone. In one sample taken from a bone graft that was about to be placed in a patient, they found 54 different pathogens. Some of these pathogens were known to be associated with conditions like pneumonia, colon cancer, leaky gut, flesh-eating bacteria, endocarditis, suppressed liver function and immune system, to name a few.

In recent news, the Hollywood icon, Dick Van Dyke, spoke of his suspicion of his dental titanium implants causing neurological problems, such as pounding headaches. He had a test administered by Dr. Hal Huggins for bacteria around the implants, which revealed a predominant number of unexplained organisms. At the age of 88, rather than undergoing extensive oral surgery to remove or replace the implants, he chose to continue to work to strengthen his immune system to address the additional body burden of the bacteria and galvanic reactions. Dick has maintained a healthy lifestyle for many decades, which has included regular exercise like swimming and rebounding. His attraction to holistic health and a positive attitude surely accounts for his youthfulness and longevity. He has recently written a book, *Keep Moving: And Other Tips and Truths About Aging*, in which he explains how he keeps mentally sharp and physically fit.

Educating the patient about the risks and benefits of any procedure is paramount to proper health care. Remember, that the implant and related galvanic reaction may become a compromise and blockage on the meridian for that tooth. I will tell the patient to stay aware of any health issues that arise that may be related to the meridian of the involved areas. It is also important for them to take action to build their immune system against the bacteria that may inhabit the area around the implant.

If after discussing my concerns about implants with the patient and the possible long-term issues, and they still decided to assume the risk, then I would refer them to an oral surgeon for extraction and implant placement. The skills of the oral surgeon are very important in maintaining the health of the bone and tissue in the long term. One particular oral surgeon would consistently do an excellent job properly preparing the extraction site for the implant, so I referred my patients to only him.

However, you can have the best oral surgeon and the best dentistry skills available, but if proper oral hygiene isn't followed, the implants may eventually cause difficulties for the patient. Under the implant crown and on the abutment, bacteria and plaque can build up if it is not attended to on a daily basis. It is extremely important that the entire area be kept clean. If a person is not willing to commit to a consistent regimen of good oral hygiene, then the implant option may not be for them.

It's pretty clear that implant dentistry is highly invasive and warrants careful consideration. It is my hope that the public is made more aware of the possible real consequences, especially for those with a body already burdened with compromising health conditions.

Using facial kinesiology to reduce anxiety

The mouth is the foundation for the expression of the face. Dentists thoroughly study the anatomy and mechanisms of the head, neck and face. We also look at the glands in the mouth that filter out the various toxins, including the tonsils and the parotid glands. We also look at the fluids of the mouth - the amount and texture can give us an indication of behavior or habits of the patient. We also study the gums or mucosa and examine the texture to see whether it is smooth or red or swollen.

Not only is the dentist looking at the anatomy for physical symptoms, we also can see indicators of emotion. For a dentist to be more effective in their work, it is helpful to be aware of the emotional state of the patient – past and present. Past emotions are often played out in facial muscles that will show a chronic emotional state. The face may look asymmetrical. For instance, a person who tends to regularly be angry or stressed, may have more developed facial muscles from bearing down on the right side. The right side of the face is the masculine, more assertive side. The left side is the creative, feminine side.

We don't need to become a therapist. For example, the dentist calls attention to the need for a splint, and the common causes for worn teeth or gum recession, and makes the observation without judgment. The patient will often understand that their anger issues are an ongoing problem. But now they see the physical manifestation of that anger, and perhaps they will do something about it.

Along with the musculature, there are neurological and energetic pathways that can be stimulated by a finger or needle. Touching an area of the head, neck and shoulders may naturally induce relaxation. If we touch the occipital muscles at the base of the skull or the trapezius muscle, the general response is relaxation. When we stimulate an area away from the mouth, it will take the patient's attention away from their mouth and pending dental procedure. The patient will often become relaxed and ready for dentistry. There is a pressure point on the palm that will help the trapezius muscles become more relaxed. It is called the Hoku Point, performed by cupping the hand and placing a thumb on the palm and applying pressure.

As I grew as a dentist, I became more aware of the mechanisms of kinesiology to enhance the dental experience of the patient. Actually, I didn't treat dental phobic patients any differently than any other patient. Everyone deserves relaxation and to be set at ease.

Is that needle sharp enough?

Because of a traumatic experience at the dentist as a child, creating the best possible dental experience for my patients has always been paramount to me.

I remember having my first toothache along with my first dental experience in the early 1940s – more than 70 years ago. This memory has stuck with me and influenced how I practiced as a dentist. It was not a good memory. My friends told me how bad it would be, and they were right.

I remember being in the dental chair as the dentist prepared the needle – and it was large. I remember that he kept his syringes in a tall glass cylinder in the corner of a small, cluttered operatory room. It was customary at that time to reuse the needles, since there were no disposables. This needle apparently required sharpening, and my dentist did it right in front of me!

This was difficult to watch, and I could see that after he sharpened the needle, he finished by aspirating the anesthetic from a small bottle into his syringe while holding it up to the window light. I thought the needle was massive, and I recall firmly squeezing the armrest of the chair when he gave me the injection. I have never forgotten this terrifying experience.

However, in the future, it did serve me, as well as my patients. When I became a dentist, I recalled that vivid memory and promised myself that I would never let the patient see the syringe. Today, with the smaller gauge and disposable needles, the injections can be administered with little or no discomfort - and there is no sharpening of the needles!

The patient is a mirror of the dentist

The dentist is an integral part of relieving anxiety in the patient. I would like to take this opportunity to share with you how I created a soothing environment and generally pleasant experience for the patient. As I mentioned before, I don't treat the dental phobic patient any differently than any other patient. It is the positive synergism of site, setting, and interaction that creates a pleasant and productive experience in the dental chair.

First, the environment itself needs to be soothing, and to promote a sense of safety and comfort. The colors in the office should not provoke or be conspicuous. We used earth tone colors throughout the office and used curves wherever possible. Curves are more gentle and calming; while sharp corners subconsciously promote anxiety.

It is also beneficial to use plants in the office. In our waiting room, we had a "living wall" that was professionally maintained to ensure the plants remained clean and bug-free. In the operatories, we would have a tree or small number of plants to create a comfortable setting. In fact, in my Westwood office, we had the same tree for more than 40 years. It was an umbrella tree named Lena, and it grew to 12 feet tall. Many of the patients saw it grow over the years and developed quite a relationship with it. Lena was an excellent source of distraction for many.

Operatories should not contribute to a claustrophobic effect of the room. It is necessary to make sure that there is no clutter in the operatory. Measures should be taken to absorb the sound of the drill so it doesn't bounce off the walls. This can be done with drapes, plants or artwork.

Another aspect of the setting is sound, which may also muffle the sound of the drill. However, it is important to not play music that is aggressive or exciting. The goal is to keep the patient's blood pressure down. The ambient music should be nonaggressive and relaxing, so it creates no physical reaction other than calming.

It is common for the dental assistant to be the one who will initially seat the patient in the operatory. The patient should be greeted with a welcome by name, a warm smile, and handshake.

The physical touch will engender a sense of comfort and welcome. The dental assistant should not discuss the procedure or finances, as it may create anxiety with the patient. The assistant should make sure that the patient is comfortable and offer a neck support and blanket. All of these initial actions set the tone that the patient's comfort is a priority.

When the dentist enters the room, the patient should be greeted again with a smile, a welcome, and a handshake. During this handshake, I would put my left hand on the trapezius and shake the patient's hand with my right hand. This would give me an indication of the patient's stress level, while it will also calm them somewhat. If this was my first visit with a patient, I would start the conversation by saying, "How may I serve you today?"

If a procedure was planned for the visit, I would ask the patient to uncross their legs, if they were crossed. This is because there is a neurological pressure point at the ankle that will block energy and blood flow, creating unnecessary stress. I would also rub the base of their skull, on the occipital muscles and move to the trapezius to promote relaxation. It also moves the focus of attention away from the mouth. The trapezius is the key to relaxation in the dental environment.

Then I would administer a few drops of Rescue Remedy, a homeopathic tincture that has a calming effect on the patient. At that time, in a very calm, gentle manner, I would say to the patient, "Give your body permission to release the old and accept the new." By creating this atmosphere of welcome, calm and comfort, the patient is usually ready to proceed.

Then came time for the injection. The patient would not ever see the needle. In fact, we would rarely allow the patient to see any of the instruments before a procedure. Everything was stored and done behind the patient.

During the injection, I would gently pull and shake the lip and tell the patient, "You will feel a little pressure." Sometimes, I even spoke to the teeth, saying something like, "Drink up, little guy." This can be distracting for the patient in a positive manner. I would then quickly withdraw the syringe and pass it to the assistant, and she would then place it out of sight.

My assistant and I would speak in soft tones, make deliberate movements, and make sure there was as little interruption as possible. This was achieved by having all of the necessary supplies readily available, plus an efficient saliva evacuation system. Interruptions are an opportunity for stress, so we would strive to have few of them. The development of an efficient and positive working relationship between the doctor and assistant can be another way to decrease patient stress.

During the procedure, both the dentist and assistant would watch the patient for signs of stress in the face and hands. The assistant would often put their hand on the patient's shoulder at times during the procedure. We would check with the patient every few minutes, to ensure they were comfortable.

In dismissing the patient, the dental assistant would remind them that an adjustment may be necessary. That would mean a short return visit to the office if the restoration had a high point that could not be addressed due to the effects of the anesthesia.

We did it the exact same way for every patient every time. All of these elements added up to a synergism of positivity and comfort. Let the healing process begin.

Chapter 10

Symptoms of Mercury Toxicity

Would you go to your dentist if you had fatigue, memory loss, tremors, or digestive issues? Probably not. Perhaps you should – if you have mercury fillings. Including a biological dentist, along with a physician, may be an effective approach in your health program.

Does every person with mercury fillings get sick? No. Does every person with mercury fillings have mercury vapor coming from those fillings? Yes.

Mercury toxicity is often very difficult to diagnose. The symptoms play out differently for different people. It depends on a person's immune system, how many other heavy metals or toxins are already in the body, genetic predisposition to mercury excretion, and many, many other factors.

Accurate testing for mercury in the body is not normally done through a simple blood, hair or urine test. Mercury is stored in the tissue, organs and fat, and it does not typically stay in the blood stream or come out in feces or urine. In fact, if mercury is detected in the urine or hair, it often means that person is a good "excreter" and is not retaining as much mercury as those who are not naturally eliminating the toxin. People who are ill from mercury toxicity are often holding onto mercury in parts of the body that are difficult to reach or test.

All forms of Mercury are toxic

Three main forms of mercury are measurable in the human body, and they are all toxic: methylmercury, ethyl-mercury, and inorganic mercury.

While methylmercury is mobile and easily absorbed, it accumulates in the tissues and is difficult for the body to eliminate. Methylmercury enters the tissue and breaks down into inorganic mercury.

Elemental mercury vapor also breaks down into inorganic mercury and accumulates in tissues. Most organic forms of mercury will eventually break down into inorganic mercury. Once inside of the tissue, inorganic mercury is very difficult to remove.

Mercury in a dental filling travels to other parts of the body in four different ways, which causes symptoms to vary from person to person. Mercury is highly volatile, evaporating from the surface at room temperature. There is no dispute that mercury vapors are emitted from mercury fillings. As mentioned in the previous chapter, the presence of gold fillings or crowns significantly raises the level of mercury vapors in the mouth and are not safe to leave under a crown. The patient will get a body-wide mercury exposure from that amalgam.

Mercury vapor is absorbed into the lungs. Because people constantly breathe, approximately 80% of mercury vapor from dental fillings is absorbed by the lungs. If a person were to stop breathing, they would decrease the amount of mercury vapors in the lungs, but other problems would quickly arise. If a person with mercury fillings chews gum for 10 minutes, the levels of mercury vapor will increase 6 to 15 times. These levels can reach as high as 100 micrograms per cubic meter. As a person chews and breathes in through their mouth, mercury vapors are inhaled and absorbed by the lungs. The blood transports the mercury to the kidneys, liver, and brain.

OSHA safe limits for mercury in the workplace is one-tenth (.10) of a microgram per cubic meter. If you were a building, you would be evacuated – if you chewed gum with mercury fillings in your teeth. Now, add eating meals, warm drinks, and grinding teeth to your daily routine, and it is a perfect scenario for chronic mercury poisoning.

Mercury vapor is picked up by nerve endings and blood vessels in the nose. Small receptors in the nerve endings in the nose absorb mercury vapors. The nerve cells containing mercury then travel into olfactory bulbs and gain easy access to other parts of the brain. Since there are a large number of arteries and veins in the area, mercury may also find its way into the bloodstream, carrying this toxic substance to the brain.

The mouth absorbs Mercury through the roots, bones, and gums. Mercury can be absorbed from the roots of the teeth, especially if there is a crown over the mercury filling.

The crown prevents the mercury from vaporizing and the mercury absorbs into the roots, gums and bones. The mercury "tattoo" is often seen on the gums surrounding a tooth with a mercury filling. Mercury fillings are a well-known cause of periodontal disease.

Mercury filling material goes into the stomach.
Microscopic pieces of mercury fillings begin to fracture away from the edges within days of placement and the surfaces immediately begin to corrode and show depletion of mercury. Mercury fillings "wear out" after approximately 12 years. Some studies say as many as 15 years, while others say as few as 8 years. Regardless of the lifespan of the amalgam filling, replacing it again with mercury amalgam starts the process of corrosion and vaporization all over again and creates extremely high levels of mercury vapors during the replacement process. Once the mercury and other metals are in the stomach, the blood stream can lead them to other areas of the body.

Mercury fillings affect the body in a chronic way, a small amount of mercury is continually absorbed into the body over a period of years. Accumulation of mercury in the body may result in permanent damage to the nervous system, brain, heart, kidneys, lungs, and immune system.

Mercury from top to bottom

Mercury fillings aren't the only source of mercury exposure to humans. The EPA has a good explanation about how humans are exposed to mercury, all the way from air to fish:

"Mercury in the air eventually settles into water or onto land where it can be washed into water. Once deposited, certain microorganisms can change it into methylmercury, a highly toxic form that builds up in fish, shellfish and animals that eat fish. Fish and shellfish are the main sources of methylmercury exposure to humans. Methylmercury builds up more in some types of fish and shellfish than others. The levels of methylmercury in fish and shellfish depend on what they eat, how long they live and how high they are in the food chain."

Mercury in fish and seafood

We know that certain seafood items can be an important food source of omega-3 fatty acids. Many of us may question purchasing seafood after the recent news that 84 percent of fish worldwide is too high in mercury. Species of fish – such as marlin, tuna, shark, swordfish, king mackerel, tilefish (Gulf of Mexico), and northern pike – that are long-lived and high on the food chain – contain higher concentrations of mercury than others.

It is also essential to be aware of the PCB levels in fish, since this contaminant has serious long-term effects. When ordering fish in a restaurant or buying it at the market, be sure to inquire about the source of the fish or seafood. Farm-raised fish tends to be high in PCBs and antibiotics.

My suggestion is to only shop where you can find out where the fish or seafood was caught, then research that location and fish species for contamination levels and warnings. If you are a sushi aficionado, be extra careful about sources and fish types, since regular consumption of contaminated fish could be very harmful. Because contamination levels can change frequently due to pollution and spills, it is best to check your sources on a regular basis.

Other sources of Mercury

Here is a list of the most common forms of mercury exposure due to human activity. This is not a complete list, but it will give you an idea of how pervasive this toxin is in our everyday life.

> Combustion of fossil fuels (especially coal)
> Electricity-generating power stations
> Gold and mercury mining
> Manufacture of cement, pesticides, chlorine, caustic soda, mirrors, and medical equipment
> Industrial leaks
> Dentistry: amalgam waste
> Corpse incineration (cremation of amalgams)

Common Products Containing Mercury

Flu shot and Vaccines, when typically delivered from multi-dose vials, which can be found as "thimerosal" – also in ear drops and nose drops. Check manufacturer label before receiving any vaccine or flu shot.

Antiques - clocks, barometers and mirrors

Button Cell Batteries - approximately 2.5 – 10.8 mg of mercury

Water-Based Latex Paint – although mercury was discontinued in 1991, remodeling activities may increase exposure

Skin-Lightening Creams - Check the label of any skin lightening, anti-aging or other skin product. If you see the words "mercurous chloride," "calomel," "mercuric," "mercurio," or "mercury," stop using the product immediately.

Non-Electronic thermostats

Fluorescent Lights
  • Fluorescent light tubes contain 4 to 50 mg each.
  • Compact fluorescent light bulbs contain approximately 4 to 8 mg each

Switches and Relays

Connecting symptoms to cause

You will notice the list of symptoms is very extensive, and it can be hard to believe that mercury toxicity causes it all. The problem is that physicians rarely consider or diagnose heavy metal toxicity when a patient presents some of these symptoms. Each person handles toxicity differently. The mercury may be held in a different part of the body than the next person, or they are already compromised with other illness or other heavy metals or toxins. This is part of the reason why mercury toxicity is very difficult to diagnose. However, when a patient's symptoms cannot be identified with another condition or illness, then heavy metal toxicity should be explored.

Here is a list of symptoms of mercury toxicity.

Psychological Symptoms
Restlessness
Anxiety/nervousness, often with difficulty in breathing
Irritability

Emotional instability: lack of self-control, fits of anger, with violent, irrational behavior
Exaggerated response to stimulation
Fearfulness
Loss of self confidence
Indecision
Shyness or timidity, being easily embarrassed
Short-term memory loss
Inability to concentrate
Mental depression, despondency
Withdrawal
Suicidal tendencies
Manic depression
Insomnia
Lethargy/drowsiness

Central Nervous System Conditions
Numbness and tingling of hands, feet, fingers, toes, or lips
Muscle weakness progressing to paralysis
Tremors - trembling of hands, feet, lips, eyelids or tongue
Myo-neural transmission failure resembling Myasthenia Gravis
Motor neuron disease (ALS)
Multiple Sclerosis
Fibromyalgia
Incoordination
Ataxia - loss of full control of bodily movements

Head, Neck and Oral Cavity Disorders
Bleeding gums
Alveolar bone loss
Loosening of teeth
Excessive salivation
Bad breath
Metallic taste
Burning sensation, with tingling of lips, face
Tissue pigmentation (amalgam tattoo of gums)
Leukoplakia
Stomatitis (sores in the mouth)
Ulceration of gingiva, palate, tongue
Dizziness - acute, chronic vertigo
Tinnitus - ringing in the ears
Hearing difficulties
Speech and visual impairment – glaucoma, restricted, dim vision

Systemic Effects
Allergies
Chronic headaches
Severe dermatitis
Unexplained reactivity
Thyroid disturbance
Subnormal body temperature
Cold, clammy skin, especially hands and feet
Excessive perspiration, w/frequent night sweats
Unexplained sensory symptoms, including pain
Unexplained numbness or burning sensations
Unexplained anemia -G-6-PD deficiency
Chronic kidney disease - nephrotic syndrome, renal
dialysis, kidney infection
Adrenal disease
General fatigue
Loss of appetite/with or without weight loss
Loss of weight
Hypoglycemia

Immunological Symptoms
Repeated infections: viral and fungal, mycobacteria,
candida and other yeast infections
Cancer
Autoimmune disorder
   -arthritis
   -lupus erythematosus (LE)
   -multiple sclerosis (MS)
   -scleroderma
   -amyolateral sclerosis (ALS)
   -hypothyroidism

Cardiovascular Effects
Abnormal heart rhythm
Characteristic findings on EKG: abnormal changes in the
S-T segment and/or lower broadened P wave
Unexplained elevated serum triglyceride
Unexplained elevated cholesterol
Abnormal blood pressure, either high or low

Gastrointestinal Effects
Food sensitivities, especially to milk and eggs
Abdominal cramps, colitis, diverticulitis
Chronic diarrhea/constipation

Endocrine and Reproductive Effects, including pituitary, thyroid and adrenals
Adverse effects on developing fetus, sperm and male reproductive organs
Spontaneous abortions or stillbirths

Again, this list is extensive and may seem like mercury toxicity can be blamed for most any condition. However, each person reacts differently, depending on susceptibility, genetic predisposition, other toxins, and many other factors. There is no one set of symptoms that point only to mercury toxicity, which is why mercury toxicity remains largely undiagnosed.

Proceed with caution

All of the chemical reactions associated with the mercury molecule - its complexity and ability to synergize with other chemicals in the body - can cause a general interruption of body function, depending upon the factors of health, nutrition, genetics, and psychological condition. These components play into the outset of disease.

A seemingly healthy person who would like to remove mercury fillings can usually do so without much difficulty, provided that the dentist follows safety protocols. But when a person is already compromised in the liver, kidneys, or neurologically, it is prudent for the dentist to work closely with a physician to determine the specific mercury removal and detoxification process, also referred to as the team approach. The physician prepares the patient prior to the removal of the mercury from the mouth, by strengthening weakened organs or immune system. Then, when the patient is ready, the mercury removal may proceed.

Testing for Mercury toxicity

Over the years, methods for determining levels of mercury in the body have been under development. The most effective tests are not typically available through a general physician. It is necessary to seek out holistic physicians who understand the effects of heavy metal toxicity. Because mercury hides in the tissues, it needs to be forced out to be measured. This is an evolving field, so it is important to research available testing methods and decide which one is right for you.

For example, one of the testing methods is called DMPS and DMSA. It is also called a Mercury Challenge Test. In simple terms, DMPS (taken intravenously) and DMSA (taken orally) are sulfite salts (dipropyl methane sulfonamide salts) used to pull the mercury out of hiding places and into urine and/or feces. They are then collected and analyzed to determine the amount of heavy metal toxicity in an individual. When I took my Mercury Challenge Test, the lab report showed my mercury levels as literally going off the page; while previous blood tests did not show mercury in my system. Since then, the DMPS protocols for challenging and chelating mercury have been found to have some adverse effects, so many health professionals have moved away from this method.

In recent years, another mercury test was developed by Christopher Shade, PhD. Mercury speciation is an analytical testing process that separates and measures the different forms (species) of mercury present in a test sample. The speciation analysis measures the biologically available forms of mercury (methylmercury and inorganic mercury). Speciation testing differs from conventional "total" mercury analysis. Rather than simply delivering an undifferentiated lump-sum total, speciation of mercury provides important data on the ratio of methylmercury to inorganic mercury. In addition, the mercury measurement process can be expanded to include rare forms of this toxic element (ethylmercury and propylmercury). From the test results, more personalized detoxification methods may be administered.

All dentists are Mercury toxic

After looking at all of the symptoms of mercury toxicity, one might think we are all mercury toxic. Most of us are probably mercury toxic to some degree. But all dentists are certainly mercury toxic. Even dentists who don't place mercury fillings are still exposed to mercury during the removal process of the mercury filling. The exposure is greatly minimized if they use mercury removal safety protocols. But the average dentist in contact with the removal and/or placement of mercury fillings experiences considerable levels of exposure on a daily basis.

Autopsy studies show people with mercury fillings have toxic levels of mercury in their brain and kidneys. The half-life of mercury can last from several years to decades, as shown by the autopsy studies. A review of 32 out of 40 studies evaluated for consistency and methodology, found that those people exposed to inorganic mercury showed significant memory deficits in testing.

Mercury easily passes to the central nervous system and lodges in tissues. Case-controlled studies have shown that tremors, impaired cognitive skills and sleep disturbances were experienced by people who work in places with exposure to mercury vapor, even at low concentrations. Dentists were found to score significantly worse than a comparable control group on neuro-behavioral tests of motor speed, visual scanning, visual motor coordination, concentration, visual memory, and emotional and mood tests.

To the dental professionals and general public that have undiagnosed and unexplainable symptoms, who have been told it's all in their head, I say to you that there is hope. Mercury toxicity is very real and not so rare, and now there is something you can do about it.

Chapter 11

Wellness through Detoxification

Most of us know someone who has a physical ailment that physicians don't know the cause or how to treat. Some of these conditions include fibromyalgia, chronic fatigue, depression, and headaches. The physician resorts to giving a prescription for the symptom, in hopes it will go away. When it does not subside, they try another pill or surgery. This is mainstream, allopathic medicine. The word "detoxification" is not typically in their vocabulary.

"Alternative" medicine isn't really alternative at all. Using natural processes to heal the body is the natural thing to do. Your body strives to heal itself automatically. Too frequently, we ingest chemicals that inhibit that process or create another condition, often called a side effect. "Mainstream medicine" uses methods which may involve ingesting chemicals or cutting out body parts to address symptoms, masking the underlying cause, which may interfere with the body's natural healing process.

Chronic mercury poisoning can cause a large number of incapacitating and supposedly incurable conditions. If mercury poisoning is recognized, it can be treated and significantly alleviated. Mainstream medicine believes that mercury poisoning is rare. It is not. Heavy metal toxicity is quite common. As a result, many people who aren't aware of toxicity often suffer needlessly. When all else has failed, treating these conditions as mercury poisoning often brings considerable improvement of overall health and even recovery.

Over the years, I personally have utilized many methods commonly employed for detoxification protocol. We begin to understand detoxification once we realize that we can dislodge the toxin from its location, either through a dose-administered sulfite process like DMPS or naturally with diet, supplementation, and physical regimens. We can use various foods that also contain elements of the sulfite group that would naturally detoxify the body. Nutritional support should always accompany any kind of therapy used by medical practitioners.

Generally, before beginning a detoxification process, it is recommended to remove the source of mercury from the body, which would be the mercury dental filling. If you detoxify while the fillings are still present, that could have additional toxic consequences. Taking a thorough patient history helps to identify other mercury sources. For instance, one of my patients was a fashion model who lived on tuna sandwiches. She was highly mercury toxic without a mercury filling in her mouth. So it is prudent to first address the source.

Many individuals have had mercury toxicity from eating an abundance of highly toxic fish. Mercury in water contaminates the algae, leading to the whole food chain. Crustaceans eat the algae, small fish eat crustaceans; bigger fish eat the smaller fish, and mercury continues to accumulate. Once you add in the toxic components of the canning processes, it would not be unreasonable to be highly suspicious of the safety of that food.

By taking a comprehensive health history, we can assess the condition of the patient, and whether they are ready for mercury removal. If a patient indicates issues with the liver, kidneys or immune system – or has any significant compromise in their health – then referral to a physician is required and imperative before starting any mercury removal. I can't stress this enough. Before anyone goes through mercury removal or starts a detoxification protocol, I strongly advise them to see a physician for evaluation. Once the source of toxicity is removed, detoxification follows.

Pathways to detoxification

The choices in detoxification methods range from a basic supplementation approach done at home to a physician-supervised protocol that involves several office visits and lab work. I'll list some here, but because detoxification needs vary so greatly among people, I am not going to describe specific protocols. My intention is to discuss the concepts in detoxification, but it is up to you to get the assistance you need for your particular situation.

First, determine your toxic body burden. This should be done through tests taken under the supervision of a health professional who is familiar with detoxification. Each practitioner has developed their own approach. Find someone with whom you are comfortable and feel you could complete the program.

DMPS-DMSA diagnostic tool and therapeutic technique

One method of finding the level of mercury toxicity in the body is the DMPS Challenge Test. While new findings show that a glutathione protocol is safer and more effective for mercury testing and chelating, I will describe the DMPS protocol. As with any health program, consult your health care provider for the best method for you.

DMPS consists of administering an intravenous "push" of the DMPS chelating agent for a 5 to 15-minute period. The administration of DMPS, a sulfite solution of varying degrees, is by prescription of the practitioner. The patient collects urine samples for the next few hours, then a determination can be made as to the amount of mercury that is in the body as shown by the amount that is released.

It is not advisable to have the DMPS Challenge Test done unless a qualified physician has provided an adequate physical workup. It is important not to stress the organs of release, such as the kidneys or the liver. If the organs are already compromised, the patient may become more ill. Discernment is used in this testing period. An oral chelating agent, DMSA, may be used, which is not as extreme. It is important for the physician to have had some prior training to perform the test. It is often advised to reinforce the immune system with proper diet and supplementation.

Once the physician knows the level of toxicity, nutritional support is established. The next step is the therapeutic administration of those salts that will detoxify or chelate the toxins out of the body. In addition to drawing mercury out of the body, DMPS also draws out zinc and copper, which are beneficial minerals in the body. The physician supplements zinc and copper during detoxification. Nutritional support is established to compensate for this detoxification protocol.

Glutathione – a developing protocol in detoxification

In recent years, the development of glutathione supplements have shown to be very promising for effective mercury chelation. It is the body's chief antioxidant and main detoxifier. It is the important molecule needed to stay healthy and prevent aging and disease. Glutathione strengthens the immune system's resistance to viruses. It helps energy metabolism run efficiently and protects each cell's delicate composition. Your body produces its own glutathione. However, stress, trauma, aging, infections, pollution, toxins, medications, and radiation all deplete glutathione. A deficiency of glutathione increases susceptibility to unrestrained cell degeneration from oxidative stress, infections, free radicals, and cancer. The liver gets overloaded and impaired, making it unable to perform its most important function – detoxification.

Glutathione contains sulfur chemical groups, which makes it sticky. With healthy levels of glutathione, toxins link to it and get carried out of the body through bile and the stool.

Eating sulfur-rich foods like onions, garlic, and cruciferous vegetables (kale, broccoli, cauliflower, collards, cabbage, or watercress) can naturally boost your glutathione levels. Exercise also improves your glutathione levels, immune system and promotes detoxification. Typically, when taking glutathione orally, absorption is inhibited by breakdown in the stomach. Therefore, it is important to find a supplement proven to achieve successful absorption.

Exit doors for toxins

Understanding how toxins exit the body may also suggest ways to naturally encourage their elimination. Once the toxins are dislodged, the body releases them through: perspiration 20%; urination 20%; bowel movement 50%; and exhalation (minimal).

Since most of toxins leave the body via the colon, adequate bowel movements – twice, or at least once a day – are crucial. The facilitation of these bowel movements may be supported in several ways. Exercise, including yoga, stretching, and rebounding, naturally manipulates the body to move waste. Roughage included in the diet, such as psyllium seed products, also assists elimination. Hydrotherapy, colonics or enemas may be included. Laxatives, however, should be avoided.

Adequate water intake is also required to promote bowel evacuation. The general rule for the amount of water to drink in a day is half of one's body weight in ounces. So, a person who weighs 150 pounds, should drink at least 75 ounces a day. This does not include the liquid from teas, coffees, colas, etc. Avoid caffeine, nicotine, aspartame and other sugar substitutes. An acceptable natural sweetener would be a naturally processed stevia.

Detoxification should be accompanied by perspiration. Using a sauna is an excellent way to sweat out toxins. In my early toxic days, I could not tolerate being in a sauna for a long period of time. I would get headaches as a result of dislodging the toxins. I started with sitz baths. I drew a hot bath with Epsom salts, creating a hypertonic solution that would draw out some of the fluids, including the toxic fluids of my body.

After periodic sitz baths, I graduated to short intervals in the sauna. I grew to enjoy the heat. If you don't enjoy the heat, the infrared sauna may be preferable, since it allows you to attain perspiration quicker. For more than twenty years, I have taken a prolonged sauna approximately twice a week.

Detoxification through colon cleansing

Stimulating the colon and keeping it clean through use of natural fibers of the vegetable kingdom, grains, flax, psyllium seed promote natural detoxification.

As a child, I was familiar with the concept of colonic irrigation by way of the enema. My grandfather was from a small town in Sicily, was trained in alternative healing processes through a sort of mysticism, for which the cleansing of the colon through enemas was a common remedy. My grandfather suggested to my mother the use of enemas to help my constipation as a child. This early exposure helped me to be open to the idea of colon cleansing.

To this day, my strong commitment to saunas and regular colon cleansing has resulted in the construction of a sauna with a clinical colonic machine as a part of any home I have owned for the past 25 years. My natural allegiance to performing colonics while taking a long sauna session has greatly contributed to my recovery and longevity, as a dentist and a human being.

I'm hungry! What's for dinner? - Detoxification with food

I used the DMPS Challenge as a means of detoxifying and monitoring progress, along with natural methods of detoxifying, including diet. I took daily supplementations of chlorella, spirulina, green algae, cilantro, and garlic. I also avoided fish and seafood with high amounts of mercury.

Green foods are natural detoxifiers and will act as scavengers while toxins are circulating in the system, increasing oxygen content, and purifying the blood. They are the essential building blocks of any healthy and vibrant diet. The active detoxifying ingredient is chlorophyll, which rids the body of environmental toxins, heavy metals, herbicides, and pesticides. Chlorophyll is found in leafy greens, broccoli, cucumbers, celery, sprouts, dandelion teas, and chlorella supplements.

Dehydrated green products can be very useful; however, live food is always best. We all have busy lives, and if we have to forego live food because of time restraints, availability or convenience, then a powdered green product is better than not having any green at all. It is important to discern the quality of any of the dehydrated green foods or drinks. The most common ingredients in green drinks are chlorella, spirulina, green algae, cilantro, wheat grass, probiotics, antioxidants, minerals, sea foods, and dark green foods. Stay away from green drinks with artificial sweeteners. Natural sweeteners like stevia can make the difference in a good-tasting green drink.

There are many brands available, but the very best green drink is the one that you are taking every day. Choose one that tastes good to you. If you commit yourself to using a quality green drink formula, every single day for 30 days, it is likely that you will be using green drinks for the rest of your life. This consistent supplementation of important detoxifiers can provide other body benefits and a feeling of wellbeing – a much better feeling than you get from a candy bar.

Here is a list of some of the other foods that promote natural detoxification:

Beets - Full of nutrients, good source of vitamins B3, B6 and C, plus beta-carotene, magnesium, calcium, zinc, and iron. Besides detoxification, the fiber is great for digestion and elimination.

Lemons – They stimulate the liver and purify our blood. They also promote digestion by increasing the release of enzymes. Vitamin C helps convert toxins into a water-soluble form that can be easily eliminated from the body. Lemon is a citrus fruit, but when lemon juice has been fully metabolized and its minerals dissociated in the bloodstream, its effect is alkalizing and raises the pH of body tissue. Sipping a small amount of warm lemon water throughout the day, helps to mineralize the body and lymph. But don't forget a straw! This protects the teeth's enamel from the lemon. Also, more is not better. Too much lemon may cause dehydration, arthritis or osteoporosis.

Apples - The soluble fiber in apples, pectin, is helpful in removing heavy metals and food additives from our bodies. It stimulates bile production, which the liver uses to release toxins. Apples include a lot of fiber and nutrients. Be sure to eat only organic apples. Conventional apples are heavily-sprayed with pesticides.

Artichokes – They increase bile production and purify and protect the liver. They also have a mild diuretic effect on the kidneys, which aides in toxin removal once the liver breaks them down. They are also very high in fiber, which helps with elimination.

Garlic - Raw garlic stimulates the liver into producing detoxification enzymes that help filter toxins from the digestive system. It also has powerful antiviral, antiseptic and antibiotic properties.

Green Tea – This is a good source of antioxidants, including catechins, which increase liver function.

Lentils and beans – They are good sources of zinc, which boosts the immune system that the body needs for normal metabolic processes in all your organs. Zinc is also key to many biochemical processes that aid in digestion and liver metabolism and is important to supplement during a DMPS protocol.

Eggs - Sulfur is found in raw and soft-cooked egg yolks, and is needed for detoxification pathways in the liver, and to bind toxic metals. Raw eggs may be consumed, but they contain avidin, a minor toxin, and sometimes the eggs contain harmful bacteria. It is recommended that you have soft-boiled eggs cooked for up to about three minutes, poached eggs, or very lightly fried eggs or very soft scrambled eggs only.

For many years, my morning routine before going to the dental office included a fiber formula in 10 ounces of water and some live probiotics before my shower. Then during my morning drive to work, I enjoyed a protein drink blended with a green powder, raw egg, and stevia. On the weekend, my favorite healthy breakfast consists of oatmeal with butter and two soft-boiled eggs on top.

Dr. Huggins suggested this delicious and beneficial meal many years ago.

Lymph – the other circulatory system

Most people only become aware of the lymph system in the context of cancer. It is widely regarded as a lesser sister to the circulatory system. However, the lymphatic system is a crucial participant in your body's ability to heal from injury and ward off disease. The lymphatic system works quietly behind the scenes to clean up the mess made by practically all of the other systems of the body.

In Europe and Far Eastern countries, the lymphatic system is recognized by doctors for its importance in preventive health care, and for how its function supports every other system in the body, including the immune, digestive, detoxification and nervous systems.

In America, we often boast about our advances in health care and research, but our practitioners don't think much about the lymph system until something goes wrong. When infection causes a swollen lymph node, or when we develop cancer in a lymph gland, or cancer elsewhere that metastasizes through the lymph vessels, then evaluation of the lymphatic system begins.

The reality is that the body has two times as much lymph fluid as blood. The lymph continuously bathes each cell and drains away waste and toxins in a circulatory system powered only by breathing and movement. You would die in a matter of hours, if the movement of the lymph completely stopped.

Lymph is about 95% water. Without adequate water, lymphatic fluid cannot flow properly. One of the most common causes of lymph congestion is dehydration. Only water can adequately rehydrate the body.

As I mentioned, exercise and body movement circulate lymph. Aerobic exercises are wonderful for sweat and bringing oxygen into the system. Most physical exercise will accomplish this. However, Bouncercise or rebounding on a small trampoline for 10 to 25 minutes is one of the easiest and most effective ways to pump the lymph, with low impact on the joints. The gentle bounce creates alternating weightlessness and double gravity to produce a pumping action that pulls out waste products from the cells and pushes oxygen and nutrition in from the bloodstream.

Massage or dry brushing also moves lymph around the body. Some massage therapists specialize in "lymphatic massage," which is a special form of massage that targets the flow of lymph in the body. It uses a certain amount of pressure and circular, rhythmic movements to stimulate the lymph. This increases its movement towards the heart for the drainage of fluid and waste. Studies have shown that lymphatic massage pushes up to 78% of stagnant lymph back into circulation. This mobilizes toxins for elimination, lessening the burden on the lymphatic system.

Practicing yoga will also encourage lymphatic circulation through movement and breathing exercises. Escalating oxygen in the blood will also increase the amount of oxygen that gets passed to the lymphatic system. Most diseases or cancer can't thrive in and around oxygenated cells. Human vitality relies on oxygenation, circulation, and good nutrition.

Unfortunately, American mainstream medicine puts a low emphasis on the lymphatic system, which is such an important process in the body. Becoming proactive in your health choices, getting educated about the body and its natural processes, and encouraging circulation and detoxification is key to optimal health and healing.

Chapter 12

"Show Me the Science"

It is now time to put the cards on the table and to show why mercury fillings should be banned from dentistry. In this chapter, I'll do my best to present research from each side of the mercury dental amalgam filling issue. We will compare the official positions of the American Dental Association (ADA) and the International Academy of Oral Medicine and Toxicology (IAOMT), and the associated research to support those positions. I will also comment on the positions to help clarify them and add perspective.

Official Position of the Use of Mercury Dental Amalgam -ADA:

"Dental amalgam serves as a safe, durable and affordable material in restorative dentistry. However, the fact that its formulation includes mercury has raised safety concerns in the minds of some. Small amounts of mercury vapor can be released from amalgam during placement, mastication and brushing.

The safety of dental amalgam has been studied and reviewed extensively, and no association has been found between amalgam restorations and any adverse health effects. The U.S. Food & Drug Administration, the U.S. Environmental Protection Agency and the Centers for Disease Control and Prevention all support the safety of dental amalgam. In addition, a European Commission scientific committee has concluded that "current scientific evidence does not preclude the use of amalgam or alternative materials in dental treatment."

Official Position of the Use of Mercury Dental Amalgam - IAOMT:

"The IAOMT seeks a ban on the use of encapsulated mercury fillings as a dental restorative material. The risk of illness or injury associated with the use of dental mercury presents an unreasonable, direct and substantial danger to the health of dental patients as well as dental personnel. Mercury fillings potentially endanger the health of individuals who have been or will be exposed to dental mercury. The weight of the published scientific evidence decidedly supports the position of the IAOMT."

The ADA acknowledges that mercury vapor is released from its dental amalgam in the statement – an accomplishment in itself. Though the concern was raised more than 100 years ago, the ADA did not admit it publicly until 1984.

Let's look at the statement, "Small amounts of mercury vapor can be released from amalgam during placement, mastication and brushing." The average filling contains 300 mg of mercury, and releases an average of 13 micrograms per day. That is just one filling. Most people have multiple mercury fillings. It is important to consider that we are chewing throughout each day, and hopefully brushing our teeth at least once daily. Because of this, logically, isn't mercury exposure worth serious consideration and exhaustive research? Where does the mercury go when chewing gum or food? As mentioned, 80% of mercury vapor is absorbed in the lungs, where the blood transports it to the kidneys, liver, and brain.

The ADA is very selective about the scientific "research" used to show that mercury fillings are safe. Because dental amalgam has been around for so long, the FDA grandfathered it in. It is impossible to prove mercury is not toxic and that mercury vapor does not release from the dental amalgam through industry-standard, clinical trials. The ADA's most consistent message is that mercury fillings have been used for more than 150 years, so they must be okay.

The IAOMT's position is pretty clear. In their view, there is a great quantity of scientific evidence showing the serious risks involved in the use of mercury in dentistry to patients and dental personnel, so it should be banned.

Both sides cite supporting evidence for their positions. Let us take a closer look.

ADA Supporting Evidence #1:
2006 Studies on effects of mercury release on children

This is their best evidence. It is the one that they frequently cite to prove that amalgam is safe. The text below is from the ADA website; I have broken it apart to make it easier to read and understand.

"In 2006, the Journal of the American Medical Association (JAMA) and Environmental Health Perspectives published the results of two independent clinical trials designed to examine the effects of mercury release from amalgam on the central and peripheral nervous systems and kidney function.

The authors concluded that "there were no statistically significant differences in adverse neuropsychological or renal effects observed over the 5-year period in children whose caries are restored using dental amalgam or composite materials" and

"Children who received dental restorative treatment with amalgam did not, on average, have statistically significant differences in neurobehavioral assessments or in nerve conduction velocity when compared with children who received resin composite materials without amalgam.

These findings, combined with the trend of higher treatment need later among those receiving composite, suggest that amalgam should remain a viable dental restorative option for children."

Here is an extremely important sentence in this statement: "Children who received dental restorative treatment with amalgam did not, on average, have statistically significant differences ..." The words "on average" are part of the misrepresentation of the raw data of the study.

The study measured mercury in urine, porphyrins, kidney damage, and neurological damage. Mark Geier, MD, PhD, a research scientist who studies chronic illnesses also analyzed the raw data and every aspect of the study. He found the results actually revealed a significant negative impact on each of the measurements, dependent on the dosage of mercury from dental amalgams. An increase in the number and size of mercury fillings that a child had, resulted in a higher reading in urinary mercury and mercury-associated porphyrins. It also showed ongoing damage at the levels of the kidney proximal tubules. Chronic damage to the kidney proximal tubules is associated to chronic kidney disease, which is the primary type of kidney disease in the United States.

If the raw data actually showed all this damage, why does the statement say there was no significant difference in the findings? Two words: "on average." This is where the numbers are misrepresented.

The study was split into two groups: mercury amalgam and composite. Each group was then further differentiated by boys and girls. They did not differentiate by the dose of mercury, which is the amount of dental amalgam in the mouth of each child. This would be a very significant factor in relationship to the results of the effects of mercury exposure.

The original researchers averaged all of the results, concluding there wasn't much movement at all. But upon a closer examination by Dr. Geier, utilizing methods of scientific evaluation, it was consistent that the more mercury that was in the mouth, the more damage was done to the body. The compilation of data resulted in a range for each group. At the top of each range, when a subject showed a high level of mercury or kidney damage, it was directly related to a greater number of mercury fillings. Averaging these results is misleading and unscientific. The high correlation of presence of mercury and kidney damage with the amount of mercury fillings is an important finding.

Boyd Haley, PhD, Professor and Chair, Department of Chemistry at the University of Kentucky, further reveals additional important issues and findings in the study which the ADA neglects to mention. He points out that one set of participants of the study were located in Lisbon, Portugal, which is a seaport city. The diets of the children in Lisbon would be very high in fish, which also contain methylmercury. This raises an obvious concern about why this location was chosen since the mercury exposure is already very high.

Dr. Haley further states the results showed significantly less urinary excretion of mercury by the boys. This means that the mercury is still in their bodies. This is an interesting result, considering that the rate of autism in boys is four times higher than girls. One of the reasons that boys may retain mercury more or are affected more than girls is because mercury is a hormone-dependent neurotoxin. Testosterone and mercury combine to create a toxic neurochemical. Studies have shown estrogen to reduce the effect of mercury, offering some degree of protective effect.

In effect, the study the ADA holds up as prime evidence of the safety of mercury fillings, actually shows ongoing mercury toxicity damage directly related to the amount of fillings.

At this point, my scientific mind naturally wonders, if mercury is a hormone-dependent neurotoxin, what about possible correlations to prostate cancer? It seems that numerous studies would be appropriate to explore diseases in the context of mercury exposure. We all know someone who has been affected by prostate cancer, including yours truly. It is my opinion that my condition is likely to be the result of chronic mercury exposure over several decades.

ADA Supporting Evidence #2:
2011 Studies on effects of prenatal mercury exposure from maternal dental amalgam

The purpose of this study was "To determine if prenatal mercury vapor exposure from maternal dental amalgam is associated with adverse effects to cognition and development in children."

The ADA uses only this sentence from the conclusion of the study: "We found no evidence of an association between our primary exposure metric, amalgam surfaces, and neurodevelopmental endpoints."

The second sentence of the conclusion is completely ignored: "Secondary analyses using occlusal points supported these findings, but suggested the possibility of an adverse association with the (mental development indices) MDI for girls at 9 months. Given the continued widespread use of dental amalgam, we believe additional prospective studies to clarify this issue are a priority."

This study warns of a priority to research the potential risk of dental amalgam to girls' mental development indices at 9 months. Does anyone see a red flag here? This is another instance where the ADA uses a study as if it were a strong case to continue the use of mercury in dentistry – and, really, it is not.

ADA Supporting Evidence #3:
2003 paper published in the New England Journal of Medicine shows no relation between mercury and degenerative diseases

The following is another statement that the ADA often refers to regarding the safety of dental amalgam. It is on the page on the ADA.org website entitled, "Statement on Dental Amalgam":

> "A 2003 paper published in the New England Journal of Medicine states, 'Patients who have questions about the potential relation between mercury and degenerative diseases can be assured that the available evidence shows no connection.'"

The specific article they are referring to is entitled, "The Toxicology of Mercury — Current Exposures and Clinical Manifestations." If you actually read the entire article, it also makes the following statements:

> "Dental amalgams emit mercury vapor that is inhaled and absorbed into the bloodstream. Dentists and anyone with an amalgam filling are exposed to this form of mercury."

> "... amalgam fillings are the chief source of exposure to mercury vapor in the general population. Brain, blood, and urinary concentrations correlate with the number of amalgam surfaces present."

> "It has been estimated that 10 amalgam surfaces would raise urinary concentrations by 1 µg of mercury per liter, roughly doubling the background concentrations. Higher urinary concentrations are found in persons who chew a great deal."

> "Today's occupational exposures, such as in the dental office, are lower and may lead to mild, reversible effects on the kidney or mild cognitive changes and memory loss."

> "Speculation has been most intense with respect to Alzheimer's disease after a report that the brains of patients with Alzheimer's disease had elevated mercury concentrations."

"… in vitro studies have indicated that mercury can affect the biochemical processes believed to be involved in Alzheimer's disease."

In general, the article says the mercury exposure in dental amalgam is not significant, but don't take it out, because "the process of removal generates mercury vapor and that blood concentrations will subsequently rise substantially before they eventually decline."

Do any of the above statements raise a red flag to you? The ADA picked out a sentence that says there is no connection to degenerative diseases.

The authors of this article missed the thousands of studies that link mercury vapor exposure to degenerative diseases. Even the main author of this article, Thomas W. Clarkson, in previously published research entitled "The Prediction of Intake of Mercury Vapor from Amalgams" found the daily intake of mercury vapor from amalgams to be 1.6 – 15.7 micrograms during eating or chewing and a total intake of 2.5 – 17.5 micrograms per day. This is considerable daily, chronic exposure to mercury vapor. Why put mercury in the tooth to begin with?

ADA Supporting Evidence #4:
February 1999 issue of the Journal of the American Dental Association, researchers report finding no significant association of Alzheimer's Disease

Another item in the ADA Statement on Dental Amalgam states:

"In an article published in the February 1999 issue of the Journal of the American Dental Association, researchers report finding "no significant association of Alzheimer's Disease with the number, surface area or history of having dental amalgam restorations" and 'no statistically significant differences in brain mercury levels between subjects with Alzheimer's Disease and control subjects.'"

An interview with Boyd Haley PhD, revealed that the study referenced was performed by a dentist in conjunction with a research scientist who had previously worked with Alzheimer's disease and heavy metal correlation studies. In an autopsy, they compared the brain tissue of people that had Alzheimer's disease with the brains of people who did not. However, during the calculation of the data, the researchers used what is called the Bonferroni Correction. This is a way to manipulate data to make the concentration of one metal look less significant in relation to other metals. Simply comparing the levels of mercury in each brain group, produces more accurate data. In the scientific research environment, it would have been well known that the Bonferroni Correction will create the results the ADA desired: no correlation of mercury levels to Alzheimer's disease.

Dr. Haley added that, one of the graduate students who worked on this study, and whose name appears on the research document, was not shown the final paper before it was published and strongly disagrees with its findings.

No conclusive studies that show that mercury amalgams are safe, because they are not.

We could go on, but for the sake of brevity, please note the pattern here. In my opinion, there is a thread of ongoing minimization of the risks of mercury exposure. The reality is that the effects of mercury fillings have been thoroughly studied. Thousands of studies have been performed worldwide. The ADA basically maintains that any adverse result in any study is just a coincidence and no matter what anyone says, amalgam is safe because they say it is safe.

Now let us look at the evidence commonly presented by the International Academy of Oral Medicine and Toxicology (IAOMT). The motto for the IAOMT, an organization of biological dentists and health professionals, is "Show me the Science." If scientific evidence were to support the position that the use of mercury fillings were not a serious risk to health and the environment, then that would be the position the IAOMT would take. Unfortunately, the science shows otherwise, and always has. It was this philosophy that drew me to the IAOMT. It was my desire to follow the science, wherever it may lead.

IAOMT Supporting Evidence #1:
Dental "silver" tooth fillings: a source of mercury exposure revealed by whole-body image scan and tissue analysis

This well-known study is called the Vimy-Lorsheider Amalgam Sheep Studies, which was profiled on the British television show *Panorama* and the US television news show *60 Minutes*. The experiment consisted of placing 12 radioactive mercury amalgam fillings in the mouth of a sheep. The radioactive isotope would allow the mercury to be detectable if it moved to other parts of the body. After 29 days, the mercury fillings were removed from the sheep's mouth, and the entire sheep's body was scanned. The results were stunning. It clearly showed mercury in the digestive tract, kidneys, gums and alveolar bone, and liver.

> "The results of this study clearly demonstrate that substantial quantities of Hg from amalgam will appear in various body tissues as early as 29 days after placement of amalgam fillings in teeth. This Hg can be readily visualized by scintigraphy and can be easily quantified by analysis of tissue radioactivity.
>
> The experimental design of this in vivo isotope study has the advantage that all of the Hg measured originates only from dental amalgam and cannot be attributed to food, water, or background environmental sources."

The dental profession establishment responded with criticizing remarks about how sheep eat and chew very differently from humans. The critics also said environmental factors, such as mercury in the diet, were not controlled. However, the experiment was designed to look for radioactivity; not mercury. There is no radioactive mercury in nature, so any radioactivity found in the scan could have only come from the mercury fillings.

The design of the experiment was to show the "exacerbated case." There would be no further controversy about the use of mercury fillings if the scan of the sheep showed no spread of mercury from amalgam in an animal that was known for excessive chewing.

However, to further address the concerns of the dental community, a second experiment was performed – on a monkey. Primates have comparable chewing habits as humans and eat similar food. The results were essentially identical to those found with the sheep. The radioactive mercury had spread around the monkey's body in the 28-day period, which resulted in tissue concentrations quite similar to the sheep.

The findings of the monkey study were also performed and confirmed by researchers in Denmark – with the same results.

Unfortunately, to this day, it is disappointing the ADA ignores the results of the sheep and monkey studies, and certainly hasn't carried out any similar experiments.

It was these studies – along with *The Smoking Tooth* video produced by Dr. David Kennedy, which showed mercury vapor coming off of an old amalgam filling - that confirmed for me the decision to become a biological dentist.

IAOMT Supporting Evidence #2:
Maternal-fetal distribution of mercury (203 Hg) released from dental amalgam fillings

This study finds that mercury from maternal amalgam fillings can be passed to the fetus and to the breastfeeding infant. Five pregnant ewes had 12 mercury fillings containing the radioactive mercury in their teeth at 112 days gestation. Blood, amniotic fluid, feces, and urine specimens were collected at regular intervals. For a duration of 16 to 41 days after mercury amalgam placement, tissue specimens were also analyzed for radioactivity, and mercury concentrations were calculated.

> "Results demonstrate that Hg (mercury) from dental amalgam will appear in maternal and fetal blood and amniotic fluid within 2 days after placement of amalgam tooth restorations. Excretion of some of this Hg will also commence within 2 days."

All of the tissue samples examined displayed mercury accumulation. The adult experienced the highest concentrations of mercury from amalgam in the kidney and liver. In the fetus, the highest mercury concentrations appeared in liver and pituitary gland.

As the gestation period advanced, the placenta showed progressively concentrated mercury, and that milk concentration of amalgam mercury postpartum provides a potential source of mercury exposure to the newborn.

> "It is concluded that accumulation of amalgam Hg progresses in maternal and fetal tissues to a steady state with advancing gestation and is maintained. Dental amalgam usage as a tooth restorative material in pregnant women and children should be reconsidered."

Several other studies have shown that mercury in dental amalgams poses significant health risks to the mother and child. In Denmark, autopsy samples were studied from human stillbirths and early post-natal deaths. They found that the mercury concentration in the infants' kidneys, liver and cerebral cortex correlated significantly with the amount of mercury fillings in the mother. Other studies have also found that the mothers' amount of mercury amalgam significantly correlated with mercury concentration in human breast milk.

Norway, Sweden, and Denmark have banned the use of mercury fillings in dentistry; Germany and Canada have limited use for pregnant women; France, Finland, and Austria have recommended the use of alternative dental materials for pregnant women. But the ADA has continued to state that mercury fillings are safe for pregnant women and nursing mothers even though mercury clearly passes to the fetus and newborns. Again, a little mercury here and there is okay for babies, too.

IAOMT Supporting Evidence #3:
Mercury in the environment: Implications for pediatricians

A technical report by the American Academy of Pediatrics, Committee on Environmental Health, made the following statements:

> "The developing fetus and young children are thought to be disproportionately affected by mercury exposure, because many aspects of development, particularly brain maturation, can be disturbed by the presence of mercury."

> "Minimizing mercury exposure is, therefore, essential to optimal child health."

The report's conclusion states:

> "Mercury in all of its forms is toxic to the fetus and children, and efforts should be made to reduce exposure to the extent possible to pregnant women and children as well as the general population."

This report doesn't come right out and say not to place mercury fillings in children. But it says if a parent has concerns about dental amalgam, to seek out a dentist who regularly places composite fillings, because an inexperienced dentist may not properly place the composite filling, which may result in tooth loss. A dentist that places mercury fillings doesn't need to be as skilled as a mercury-free dentist.

However, throughout the report, it repeats warnings of the effects of mercury exposure to children. What is the point of placing a mercury filling in a child, if it guarantees mercury exposure to that child?

Dr. Suresh Kotagal, a pediatric neurologist at the Mayo Clinic, who also participated in the 2010 FDA Dental Products Panel meeting to discuss the health impacts of mercury amalgam fillings, very poignantly stated, "I think that there is really no place for mercury in children."

IAOMT Supporting Evidence #4:
Retrograde degeneration of neurite membrane structural integrity of nerve growth cones following in vitro exposure to mercury

In layman's terms, it means that the research explored the breakdown of neurons in the brain when they were exposed to mercury.

In a previous study, animal brains exposed to mercury vapor inhalation produced a molecular lesion in brain protein metabolism similar to lesions in 80% of Alzheimer's-diseased brains. Research scientists at the University of Calgary explored the effect of mercury on the brain further.

Under a microscope, the researchers were able to view brain neuron tissue cultures and examine how low levels of mercury ions altered the cell membrane structure of the developing neurons. No other heavy metals added at the same concentration, including cadmium, aluminum, lead, and manganese, affected the neuron. The mercury disintegrated the tubulin structure of the brain neuron.

A previous study entitled, "Brain trace elements in Alzheimer's disease" showed consistent elevated concentrations of mercury in various regions and subcellular fractions in the Alzheimer's disease brain samples. Other studies found elevated mercury in the blood and cerebrospinal fluid of Alzheimer's diseased patients.

Dr. Boyd Haley, said in another study, "The relationship of the toxic effects of mercury to exacerbation of the medical condition classified as Alzheimer's disease" explored genetic factors and exposures to mercury and other heavy metals as related to Alzheimer's disease.

Remarkable remarks

Boyd Haley, PhD, had been previously awarded grants for more than 25 years at the University of Kentucky, funded by the National Institute of Health (NIH). However, when he pursued the subject of linking mercury to Alzheimer's disease, the NIH stopped the studies, and he has not received a grant from them since. Numerous stories involving research about mercury have been suppressed over the past several decades.

Another study found that in the 1999-2000 period, mercury was detected in the blood of 2 percent of women aged 18 to 49. By the year 2006, that level had risen to 30 percent of women. This troubling information was documented by Dan Laks, who was the lead author of this study entitled, "Assessment of chronic mercury exposure within the U.S. population, National Health and Nutrition Examination Survey, 1999--2006."

Tens of thousands of studies worldwide have been done on mercury throughout the past 150 years. There have been just under one thousand studies that explore the effects of the mercury filling. In fact, there is an entire bibliography of more than 50,000 studies involving mercury compiled by Mats Hanson, PhD, entitled "Mercury Bibliography."

The science is there. It sufficiently supports discontinuing the use of mercury in dentistry. It will be up to the public to put pressure on the ADA, FDA and your dentist to stop using this toxic dental material.

National organizations ignore science, along with the ADA

The ADA cites the positions of many organizations supporting the use of mercury fillings, including the Alzheimer's Association, Autism Society of America, National Multiple Sclerosis Society, and many more. None of these organization have done any independent research regarding mercury fillings. The ADA feeds them the same manipulated studies.

As an example, the Alzheimer's Association does not do studies on mercury, a known neurotoxin that affects the brain and produces effects similar to symptoms in Alzheimer's Disease.

Let me say that again.

The Alzheimer's Association does not study mercury. I find that remarkable. In fact, if you do a search in the research section of their website, www.alz.org, for the word "mercury," no results come up. The only time they mention mercury is to repeat the position of the ADA. Aren't they curious about a possible correlation of mercury to the disease they claim to want to cure?

Precautionary Principle

The definition of the precautionary principle in the context of risk management states, "that if an action or policy has a suspected risk of causing harm to the public or to the environment, in the absence of scientific consensus that the action or policy is not harmful, the burden of proof that it is not harmful falls on those taking an action."

Neither the ADA nor the amalgam manufacturers have not been required to prove the safety of mercury fillings. Norway, Sweden, and Denmark banned the use of mercury in dentistry based on the Precautionary Principal. In the context of dental amalgam, the FDA rejects this concept of requiring proof of safety before continuing use on the general public.

I believe that there is a social and moral responsibility to protect society from exposure to harm, especially when scientific research has found there to be a plausible risk. Mercury fillings are a clear cause for great concern. They should be banned because of the existing scientific evidence. There is a definite need for additional non-biased studies to be done.

Chapter 13

Mercury Fillings Awareness: Past, Present & Future

Mercury fillings will eventually be banned. It will no longer be necessary to make consumers and dentists aware of the dangers of having a mercury filling placed. We will only need to educate dentists about the safe removal of the mercury. In the meantime, we need to increase awareness of the other facets of the dental mercury issue.

The American Dental Association has a multi-million dollar advertising and lobbying budget. As a result, they have controlled the public narrative for a long time. In fact, before 2009, their annual lobbying budget was about $400,000 per year. In 2009, it soared to $1.6 million and has held steady at about $2.5 million every year since. It has been small groups and individuals with limited funds that have bravely stood up to the misinformation that has been disseminated to the public and government agencies. The tenacity of these courageous people is remarkable.

How about some good news!

In 2006, a Zogby Poll found that 76% of consumers were NOT AWARE of mercury in dental fillings. In part, thanks to the openness of the internet and persistent messaging by mercury-free dental organizations and mercury poisoned victims, there has been an increase in awareness of the contents of "silver" fillings. By 2012, a Zogby Poll found that 57% of Americans were not aware of mercury in dental fillings. This means consumer awareness has increased almost 20% in six years. We have a long way to go, but we are making progress on the awareness front.

Educating the public is a difficult task. When someone becomes aware of mercury in dental fillings, they get all excited and talk to their dentist. Then the dentist will usually tell them that silver fillings are safe and they have nothing to worry about. This is the end of the conversation.

For about twenty years, I held free seminars in my office in Los Angeles about the dangers of mercury fillings. I also lectured with our physician, Dr. Hans Gruenn, who spoke about mercury toxicity in the body. This was not a sales pitch. We did not approach attendees to schedule an appointment. This was one person speaking up and talking about the risks and effects of mercury fillings to anyone who would listen.

Until the anti-mercury groups became more vocal and increased their outreach, most people found out about the risks of mercury fillings after they were already poisoned. These people were fortunate enough to link their health condition to mercury. The number of people who are experiencing heavy metal toxicity without a proper diagnosis is likely to be alarming. Like I said, do you go to your dentist for a stomachache? Do you go to your dentist for chronic fatigue? Do you go to your dentist for tremors? Memory loss? Fits of rage?

Thanks to the availability of the internet and search engines, people are becoming more informed. The internet will be one of the biggest tools in winning the Third Amalgam War. In fact, someday, it will be called the Final Amalgam War. It is the longest one and the most hard fought, but IT WILL BE WON.

The Internet – A strange and wonderful place

The amount of information on the internet about amalgam fillings is quite comprehensive. Fortunately, many consumer websites have information for people who are looking for answers about mercury fillings. Mercury poisoning victims, consumer activist groups and mercury-free dental organizations all post these websites.

In 2005, my wife and I took over a website, TALKInternational.com. It was actually started in Canada in 1997, when the internet was relatively new to households. It was created for the purpose of sharing information between the plaintiffs in a class-action lawsuit about dental mercury. It grew to be a popular consumer website with a directory of mercury-free dentists, discussion groups, and many free resources. TALKInternational.com continues to thrive today, helping consumers find answers to questions about dental mercury and other related holistic health issues, like fluoride, vaccinations, GMOs, and more.

Dental Mercury supporters also utilize the internet. When you look up terms like "dental amalgam," "biological dentistry," and even the late "Hal Huggins," on Wikipedia, it is quite obvious that the contributors are pro-amalgam shills. There are lots of shills and trolls on the internet lurking around comment sections of news articles and blog posts about the dental mercury topic. Some of them have their own websites. I have often thought that most pro-mercury supporters on the internet are part of the disinformation agenda of some organizations that financially benefit from implanting mercury two inches away from a child's brain.

Educating the dentist

It is clear the consumer isn't going to get information about mercury fillings from their dentist. The 2012 Zogby Poll also showed only 11% of people were told by their dentist that amalgam fillings contain mostly mercury. This is not informed consent. As we mentioned previously, for decades, dentists were not even allowed to discuss the mercury content of the amalgam fillings with the patient. So we certainly cannot place blame solely on the dentist.

A ban on mercury is the only way to get most dentists who still use amalgam to stop. Many dentists are so closed minded about the issue, even science won't convince them. After a ban, though, dentists will need to learn how to remove it safely.

Mercury-free dental organizations, like the IAOMT and IABDM offer education and training on how to set up a mercury-safe operatory and perform safe mercury removal. Check the Resource section of this book to find these organizations.

Inspired from seminars I held over the years on safe mercury removal, I started an online continuing education website so dentists can learn about biological dentistry and related topics. This is another advantage of the internet, reaching people that we could not have otherwise.

Dental Schools – a great place to start

In 2012, the College of Dentistry at New York University was the first dental school to no longer teach that mercury amalgam fillings were the preferred filling material. In a letter from the Associate Dean to the students and faculty, it stated, "Beginning immediately: All treatment plans should consider alternative restorative materials other than amalgam." The letter also included other guidelines about proper disposal and environmental protections.

It's a start. This letter was in response to the UN Environmental Program World Treaty on mercury. Someone at the university could see the writing on the wall that dental mercury is going to be phased out or banned, even if only for environmental reasons.

Here's the interesting part, and it happens over and over. When someone in the mainstream takes a position that reflects negatively on the use of dental mercury, there is some type of immediate retraction. Shortly after this letter was sent out, the Dean of the College of Dentistry stated, "The NYU College of Dentistry has not stopped teaching the use of amalgam nor does it intend to do so. Further, amalgam is now and will continue to be used in our clinics whenever indicated."

I suspect that the Dean got a scathing phone call from certain powerful people in the dental profession to make sure they don't say that mercury is bad and is still an accepted dental material.

Hopefully, other schools will fall in line, and some even take it further. The ideal situation would be for all dental schools to replace amalgam courses with teaching proper handling of mercury waste in the dental office and how to safely remove mercury from the mouth.

Dental Mercury programs and documentaries

There have been some television news segments about the dangers of mercury fillings. They are often some of the most watched programs. In 1990, the news magazine program *60 Minutes* did a report on amalgam fillings. There was a huge amount of public feedback about the airing. Unfortunately, the Gulf War broke out immediately thereafter, and all of America's eyes were on the live action in the war in Iraq being played on television.

The ADA and government agencies invested large sums of money sending out letters and news releases to dentists in the United States discrediting the scientific information presented on the *60 Minutes* program. They attempted to assure dentists that since amalgam had been used for 150 years, it must be safe. They sent press releases to major media outlets and created a special program for dentists entitled, "What To Tell Your Patients When They Ask About Amalgam."

In 1994, the BBC television show, *Panorama* – a program similar to *60 Minutes* in the United States – aired a program called "Poisons in Your Mouth." On the day following the broadcast, The Times of London carried an article attacking the program, entitled, "Panorama Scare Story.' This provoked a response from the *Panorama* presenter, Tom Mangold, whose response was entitled: "We Did Not Ignore the Good News - There is None."

The *Panorama* program was supposed to rebroadcast in North America in 1994. It never was.

"Mercury Undercover" is a 2011 documentary exposing the cause and effect of the well-hidden evidence of mercury contamination as seen through the eyes of doctors, scientists, environmental experts and mercury-poisoned survivors. A link to this film may be found in our Resource section.

At about the same time this book is printed, a documentary called "Evidence of Harm" will be released. It is an extremely well done film with high production quality. One of the remarkable parts of the film is when they visually demonstrate the levels of mercury vapor in the air as an amalgam filling is being drilled out and removed from a tooth. They use very high tech mercury sensor equipment that shows the levels of mercury vapor to be 25 times the OSHA limits for mercury vapor exposure. The patient, doctor and assistant are all exposed to these levels of contamination. I highly recommend that you see this important film and make sure your dentist sees it, too.

The mercury filling controversy is actually an information and PR war. If the public fully understood the existing scientific findings, without distraction, mercury in dentistry would have been banned long ago. It's about money. It's about power. It's a shame.

Chapter 14

For Every Action, There is a Reaction

Okay, so now you know. You can't un-ring this bell. Will you ever look at a mercury filling the same? If you have mercury fillings, you may be feeling a sense of urgency right now to get those things out of your mouth. If you are a dentist reading this book, perhaps you feel differently about the way you will practice dentistry moving forward. It is my hope that sharing my experiences and this important information will help you in some way.

I am not the first person to write a book or speak out against mercury in dentistry. There have been many people alongside me in this struggle for several decades. It saddens me to think that there even has to be a struggle.

You may be asking, if mercury is so toxic, where are all the poisoned victims? Victims of mercury poisoning can be very vocal. However, many are not. They are often too sick to make the effort. Many have lost their jobs because they are unable to work. There are some people out there trying to figure why their health is declining. They may not have made the connection until the toll on their body is too great for complete recovery.

Mercury toxicity also affects the brain and behavior. Mercury poisoning has been called Mad Hatter's Disease because mercury was used in the production of hats in the 19th century. Some people with mercury toxicity may seem a little crazy. It is the biological dental offices that have compassion and patience for these people. Some mercury poisoned victims do not have the ability to join the cause. It is incumbent upon those of us that now know the truth to stand up for the victims, past, present and future.

One person can make a difference

Over the years, I have seen great strides in the dental mercury movement. They started with one person that decided to take action. That person contacted someone else, and so on. There are some real heroes in this movement, many of which have been mentioned throughout this book. But each of those people came to the table because of an experience; each unique to them.

I have seen one particular person inspire many. Anita Tibau immediately comes to mind when I think of someone that has encouraged people to do brave things and has moved mountains in this cause. An entire book could be written about her story and accomplishments. Most recently, Anita was part of a spirited group instrumental in helping the entire country of Brazil adopt mercury free dentistry. She and others have worked tirelessly to move the cause forward. Anita is a victim of dental mercury poisoning. There are those people who experience or see the injustice and cannot let it go on.

For every action, there is a reaction

The synergism of even a small action can add up to create a major effect. There will be a tipping point. The ADA and FDA can no longer ignore the public and those dentists who have bravely decided not to toe the line and parrot the misinformation the dental establishment has perpetuated for 150 years. I have listed some ways to take action, big and small. You will also be able to view continuously updated information at TALKInternational.com. Check the Resources section in this book for links and sources to the help you take action on the items mentioned below.

Become informed: Learn more about the hazards of dental mercury
A good place to start is the IAOMT position paper. They have a comprehensive response to the ADA and FDA positions on dental amalgam. You can also check the Resources section of this book to find more information.

Share your concerns about dental mercury with your dentist
Let your dentist know that the placement and unsafe practices in the removal of mercury in his dental office is not acceptable. Ask your dentist if the dental office has an amalgam separator in use.

Join an anti-dental amalgam organization
Show up, help an organization (for example, DAMS) to increase mercury awareness in your own community. These groups have various capacities of volunteer duties available.

Submit an adverse event report on mercury fillings to the FDA

Injured consumers may submit a report to the FDA when they believe they have been poisoned by dental amalgam. The FDA will respond to a public outcry. If we get enough people reporting the toxic effects of mercury fillings on their health, they have to do something about it. You should also report any health improvement that you have after safe mercury removal.

Find and use the services of Mercury-Safe dentists

Nothing gets the attention of a dentist more than getting hit in the pocketbook. If you are going to change dentists and go to a biological dentist, let your previous dentist know why you are leaving. If they hear this more than once, they are likely to look into this issue more. Here are some websites where you can find mercury-free dentists:

TALKInternational.com
IAOMT.org
IABDM.org
HolisticDental.org

Ask your benefits administrator for a cost neutral dental plan which excludes mercury fillings

Insurance companies need to hear from subscribers that they won't accept mercury fillings as a dental treatment. If your benefits administrator understands the risks of mercury fillings, then when they tell insurance companies mercury fillings are unacceptable as a preferred treatment, insurance companies will feel the pressure to change the policy.

Write a letter

Start a letter writing campaign to your congressman, dental amalgam manufacturers, the American Dental Association, the FDA, your dental insurance company, your state dental board, and any other organization or person who is part of the chain of involvement with mercury fillings. Get friends to join in!

Dental professionals: Know your rights. Demand protection from dental mercury's toxic exposures in the workplace

If you are working in a dental office that does not protect you from mercury vapors or particulate, then talk to your employer about using safety protocols established by the IAOMT. Consider wearing a mercury vapor monitoring badge to check the levels of mercury exposure you experience during a mercury filling replacement. Contact your local OSHA office if you believe you are being subjected to unsafe levels of mercury in the workplace.

Share information about mercury fillings with others
Talk to friends, family and coworkers and ask them if they are aware that "silver" fillings are at least 50% mercury. You can be sure many of them won't know. You should also make them aware that if their dentist is going to replace a mercury filling, that they should be aware that safety protocols need to be in place during the removal. Help them make an informed decision about their next dental procedure.

On social media, "Follow" and "Like" organizations working toward the ban of mercury fillings. Share their posts and make comments.

Tell your story. If you have been mercury poisoned, tell people how you found out and what you did about it. You can do that on social media, start a blog or website, or contact TALKInternational.com to have your story posted.

Have a screening party. Get a copy of the documentary "Evidence of Harm" and have a "documentary night" at your home or school, or with an organization with which you are already involved.

Donate to organizations that are actively working on the effort to ban mercury fillings
Sometimes we want to help, pitch in, and show up, but our schedules just won't allow another thing. So, empower the organizations that are doing the work! Money talks. The ADA has millions of dollars more than all the organizations combined to counteract efforts by groups that support the ban of mercury in dentistry. Let us level the playing field with more media campaigns, legal actions, research, and others.

Check your stock portfolio.
Be sure that you are not investing in companies that promote the use of mercury in dentistry or anywhere else. If you are a stockholder of such a company, show up at the shareholders meeting and ask questions about their use of mercury and its toxic health and environmental effects.

Sponsor a safe mercury filling removal – Pay it forward
Ask your biological dentist if there are any patients who cannot afford the fees to safely remove mercury fillings. Offer to pay for

part or all of the fees for someone in need. Some of us can afford to do that. And I promise, it will feel really good.

Each of the actions above are quite doable. If each of us took just one of these actions, it would make a difference in the success in banning mercury and safe mercury removal – and, yes, it will make a difference in you.

Chapter 15

One Last Word: Circulation

My initial motivation for going into dentistry was seeing my girlfriend's boss, who was a dentist, driving around in a Cadillac and living in a nice house. Yes, I do have a Cadillac and a pretty nice house. So, I guess it worked out after all.

But what I didn't plan on was developing such a deep appreciation for my profession - dentistry, which enabled me to grow intellectually and as a person. It is an honor to work in a field where compassion is an everyday thing and an asset in serving people. Dentistry also taught me about health, and I had the good fortune to learn alongside some of the greatest minds in nutrition and health, like Dr. Linus Pauling and Dr. Brugh Joy.

Along the way, I saw an injustice, and I was complicit. I now had a duty to alert people to the truth about the contents of the "silver" filling.

In this journey, I learned so much more than the fact that mercury fillings are bad. I got to experience and observe firsthand the energy system of the body, the meridian system. I have seen needles move on various scientific instruments that verified the energy flow along the meridians from the teeth to the organs and back. I saw the results of dissimilar metals in the mouth manifest in other parts of the body. I am blessed to have been shown a most intriguing and effective approach to health and wellness.

Biological dentists have been called quacks – but not by their patients. It has been done by people who feel they already know everything there is to know about the body. I have compassion for those people, too. I was one of them.

I encourage additional serious, unbiased scientific studies of the energetics of the body. If you are looking, you will see the connection. I saw it time and time again.

I have shared with you my initial experience with mercury, from the time I was a child, to the effect that mercury had on my day-to-day life as a dentist. My body has absorbed mercury from childhood and through adulthood. I have worked and played with mercury. I put it in people's mouths, and I took it out – unprotected, for decades. Because of my continual mercury exposure – accumulating to verifiable industrial toxic levels - I am always aware of the need to employ those things that will facilitate detoxification of my body.

At 81 years old, I have been diagnosed with prostate cancer, which now occupies over 75% of my prostate gland, as verified by ultrasound. It now shows signs of migrating out of the prostate and into other areas of my body. Allopathic medicine has recommended treatments that would likely affect my quality of life, with no guarantee of increasing my longevity.

I chose methods that would slow the rate of cancer progression, but still leave me with the ability and feeling of wanting to do for myself and for others.

For the past year, I chose the route of cannabis oil, also called Rick Simpson Oil. The Indica strain of marijuana containing a cannabinol called THC is processed into a thick, tarlike oil. The active ingredient apparently reacts and interferes with the mitotic division of cancerous cells. After two months of full dosage, my PSA score went down 50%. Fortunately, in California, it is perfectly legal to obtain, possess and use this oil.

I next added a regimen of ozone therapy. I bought an ozone machine and began to administer the ozone myself. This part of my treatment has given me additional energy so I can enjoy the day, mow the lawn, play with my cats, go on a weekend outing with my wife, and live as normally as possible.

The third major component to my treatment is rebounding or Bouncercise. This has kept the lymphatic system flowing, brought more oxygen into the cells of my body and released toxins. Rebounders are often used in cancer treatment clinics for that purpose. Rebounding is also included in detoxification protocols as an ally in mercury detoxification and addressing the symptoms of lethargy and fibromyalgia.

I perform the cannabis oil therapy, ozone treatment, and Bouncercise on a regular basis. I also take saunas and colonics, as I have for the past twenty years. Occasionally, because I have felt so good, I may have slacked off on the treatment. However, overall, my regimen is manageable, doable, and has produced the results I desired.

In my most recent appointment with my urologist, while performing another ultrasound, he noted that my cancer progression was minimal – surprisingly minimal. He said he would have thought that it would have progressed further since I had not taken his treatment advice.

How did this happen anyway? Is the prostate cancer due to a lifelong exposure to mercury? I don't have an answer to that, except to say that chronic mercury exposure caused a significant, ongoing burden to my immune system.

In addition to the burden of mercury in my body, performing 50 years of sit-down dentistry may have supported the presence of cancer by the stagnation of the lower back area and spine. Eighty percent of dentists leave the profession due to work-related disorders. Dentistry is a physically demanding profession with numerous occupational hazards.

I do feel that incorporating a lifestyle of ongoing detoxification modalities probably got me to age 81, which is currently 5 years past male life expectancy in the US. I give credit to a couple of decades of saunas, colonics, quality nutritional supplementation, and daily bouncing on my Freedom Spring rebounder. Most longevity physicians will tell you that those health practices likely saved me from a premature passing. All of these practices encourage circulation. Circulation is key to optimal health.

It's about taking charge of your health and making informed choices – what this book is all about.

In these last words, I hope to share some most important lessons I have learned that may go on to help others beyond my time here.

First and foremost in my life, I have seen the importance of a positive attitude and to feel positive in the healing mode. After I had severely broken my leg in an ATV accident at age 71, I found that my body healed quicker when I changed my attitude. At first, when someone asked how my broken leg was, I told them how difficult things were. But when I changed my response to, "Wonderful and healing, doing exactly what it is supposed to do." This promoted the healing process. When I reprogrammed my thinking, I reprogrammed my healing.

I now acknowledge that one of the main ingredients in my life is the application of love in all of the things that I do. Whether it is writing a book or drilling a tooth, do it with presence, respect, and compassion. My mother was instrumental in teaching me these principles.

Make time to meditate and reflect on your life.
Clarity is important in the healing process.
Embrace life's challenges, for there are lessons in them.
Release fears and expectations.
Find harmony within the conflict of life.
Give ourselves permission for the struggle to be there and to release it.
Establish your connection to the grid, to the collective consciousness.
Be of service to yourself and to others.

And lastly, circulation, circulation, circulation - in all things: the body, food, air, water, money, laughter, love, and service.

Epilogue

Dental Office Bloopers: True Stories

I cannot tell the story of my dental career without talking about Shirley Fretto, my devoted office manager of more than 40 years. Most agree that she could write a book about all the unusual experiences in our dental office. Because our office had a reputation for not being a typical dental office, this attracted some not-so-typical people and events. Shirley was on the front line, answering the phone and working at the front desk – dealing with it all firsthand. She has been the cornerstone of my dental practice, and our patients are as loyal to her as they are to me.

I asked Shirley to contribute to a couple of her most memorable experiences, which have been favorite stories of the dental staff and our families over the years. But first, to give you some background about Shirley and full disclosure, she is actually a third cousin to me. We never told the patients that we were relatives because we didn't want people to think that she was there for any other reason than the fact that she was an outstanding office manager. For the remainder of this chapter, I present to you, Shirley, my trusted friend, confidant, and family historian.

Not Your Typical Dental Office – By Shirley Fretto

My name is Shirley Fretto, and I have been Dr. Rota's Personal Assistant and Office Manager for the past forty years. I must say, this journey has been most interesting and fulfilling. I witnessed Dr. Rota, as a young dentist, become a highly respected Assistant Professor at the UCLA School of Dentistry. His reputation in the restorative field was highly renowned. It was extremely rewarding to see his interest flourish in acknowledging mercury as a highly toxic material. He was on a crusade, and I was so proud to be a part of it, as I realized how important this was to him. There's no question in my mind that if I had the chance to do it over, I absolutely would, without hesitation. It's been an incredible ride, for which I am extremely grateful and appreciative.

Many patients who contact a biological dental office are not only interested in certain aspects of a medical condition they may have, but are mainly concerned with our protocol for mercury removal. When addressing this issue, we always inform the patient that whether they have the procedure done in our office or elsewhere, there are certain guidelines that need to be followed. And more importantly, does the office provide oxygen for the patient during the procedure? Is the doctor and staff properly protected? Nine times out of ten, the patient will tell you that's why they decided to go with our office. You will find that most dental offices do not follow this protocol. Once a patient has had all their mercury fillings removed, it's imperative they follow some type of regimen to have the mercury also removed from their body. The patient should be seen by a physician who is knowledgeable and is familiar with the criteria for safe detoxification for each individual.

While being employed in a biological dental office, I found myself subjected to numerous unusual questions that would not be asked in a "normal" dental practice. I have been asked some of the following questions during an initial phone call from a new patient inquiring about our services:

"What does the doctor normally eat for dinner?"

"What religion does he practice?"

"Is your office close to the elevator shaft? I am concerned about the cables."

"Would the doctor agree to see me on the street to do an exam?"

"Is the doctor Japanese?"

This person actually argued with me that Rota was a Japanese name and that I must be mistaken. By the way, Dr. Rota is a full-blooded Italian.

It takes a lot of patience when dealing with patients on the phone and in person. When I received that first phone call, I was the initial contact representing Dr. Rota's office. What I said could either make or break the doctor, whether or not that person would schedule an appointment. Many patients had confided in me later that they selected the office based on how I handled them on the phone.

No matter how busy I might have been at the time, I would put everything aside and devote full attention to that call. It was especially important not to seem rushed or annoyed. Everyone wants to feel that they are special at that moment. Through the years, I've had several patients tell me they decided to schedule with our office because I had taken time with them and answered their questions. They admitted they had interviewed several offices before scheduling with us. When I took the time and tried to represent Dr. Rota well on that initial phone call, the reward was greater in the long run.

A Most Unusual Patient

Probably, one of the most extraordinary experiences that occurred in the dental office, was the day, a Sheik from Arabia decided to use the services of Dr. Rota. When I received a phone call from a referring doctor's office, I was informed that this was a "high profile" person, and we were told to keep the waiting room area cleared of all other patients during his appointed time. I was told the Coordinator would be calling with the requested time. It wasn't long before I received the call. At this point, I had no idea who this person was.

As I was talking to the Coordinator, I heard him say, "Stop him, don't let him go out! They haven't blocked the street yet!" I couldn't imagine with whom we were dealing.

Then the big moment happened. Two big, black limousines pulled up in front of the building carrying the Sheik, as well as the Coordinator and six bodyguards. You could imagine the fury that this created in the office building. I was getting phone calls from other tenants wanting to know if the President was coming to our office. Needless to say, it was an exciting time!

The bodyguards themselves were quite an experience. I had never seen such beautifully dressed men. They wore Armani suits and shoes that were so polished, you could easily see one's reflection. The guards were strategically placed throughout the office. One was located inside the front door and the other on the outside. I recall the first day I needed to use the restroom, I didn't realize that there were bodyguards right outside the door. When I opened the door, one was startled and asked if worked here, and if I was coming back. With that, I attempted a joke to break the tension, sort of whimpering, "I kind of live here." No reaction. Not a smile.

Dealing with the Sheik was such a different protocol than with other patients. I was told that under no circumstances was I to discuss any financial arrangements, that the Coordinator would handle everything. I particularly remember one day the Sheik was being seen after hours, and there was a bodyguard stationed in the waiting room. Without us realizing it, a member of the cleaning crew had tried to enter the suite. I have never seen someone swing into action so swiftly. Of course, I also jumped up quickly. And recognizing her as the cleaning lady, I shouted "She's okay!" The poor woman was just shaking. It was something that neither one of us will ever forget.

There was also another occasion when the Sheik decided he was going to come in after hours for an unscheduled appointment. It just so happened to be a day when the doctor was not even in the office. The Sheik's Coordinator called me and stated he was putting the Sheik in the car to come to the office. Needless to say, I panicked, as neither the doctor nor assistant was there.

I explained to the Coordinator that it would take at least an hour, if not longer, for Dr. Rota to get into the office from his home in Malibu. He told me that I should do the best I could, since the Sheik was still coming! In order to stall for more time, the Coordinator had indicated that when the Sheik arrived, I was to put him in the dental chair by walking him very slowly, back to the operatory. During this time, I must admit, the Sheik was a most generous congenial person and actually put me at ease. The Coordinator also thought I should give him some mouthwash and instruct him to rinse several times very slowly - all in an effort to buy more time.

After seven extensive visits, the Sheik's mouth was restored and he was extremely grateful to have experienced Dr. Rota's service and his expertise with Biological Dentistry. As I recall, when he was leaving the office, he exclaimed "I like you people. I will be back!"

We never discussed financial arrangements with the Sheik himself. The Coordinator would settle the bill and would only accept fees that were many, many multiples of our customary fees. We were told that the Sheik would be insulted if he were to pay any less. We didn't argue with him.

Dangers of Dental Burs

This story is not only the most embarrassing thing that ever happened to me, but it could well be the most embarrassing that could ever happen to anyone.

One day, one of the dental assistants asked if I could seat a patient in the dental chair for her. So I took the patient from the waiting room to the operatory. It is close quarters between the dental chair and the dental handpieces. Consequently, on the floor, is a rheostat, basically a foot petal the dentist uses with his foot to control the speed of the drill bur in the handpiece. As the patient went to sit in the chair, without me realizing it, I accidentally stepped on this rheostat while backing away from the dental chair. This turned on the drill, causing the drill to enter between the cheeks of my buttocks. I was completely unaware that this had happened!

When I placed the dental bib on the patient, I realized I couldn't move. I continued to make small talk with the patient while I was feeling hot and flustered, wondering why I couldn't move.

All of a sudden, the patient turned her head around and in exasperation with a loud, annoying voice said, "What are you doing?"

I attempted to keep her quiet, as I knew the doctor was close by and could hear us in the next operatory. I asked her if she could help me, as I couldn't move.

She got out of the chair and said, in a terrified voice said, "Oh my God! It's in you!"

At that moment, Dr. Rota came around the corner, drying his hands. I could tell he was perturbed, as we were making quite a disturbance.

Dr. Rota said, "Ladies, what seems to be the trouble?"

The patient quickly said, "It's in her! The drill is in her"!

Dr. Rota came around to me, took a look, shook his head, and calmly replied, "Yep, it sure is."

By now, I am totally embarrassed and cried, "Would you just take it out?!"

The doctor is now kneeling on the floor, while he gently unscrews the drill from my buttocks.

The patient started laughing hysterically and exclaimed, "I can't wait to get to my bridge club to tell everyone what just happened!"

All I wanted was to quietly disappear and not be seen again. And to top it off, Dr. Rota made me get a tetanus shot. I steered clear of the rheostat for the rest of my dental office career.

Years later, one of our employees, Scott Chavez, also taught dental assisting at a local technical school. For an icebreaker on the first day of class, he would tell my story about the dental bur incident. Well, one day, we hired a new dental assistant who had been in one of Scott's classes. When she realized this was the office in the story, she exclaimed to me, "Oh my God! You're the bur in the butt lady!"

Now, it's a favorite story often told at office parties and family gatherings. I hope to be famous for something else someday.

Recommended Resources

Biological Dentistry Organizations

International Academy of Oral Medicine & Toxicology
www.IAOMT.org

International Academy of Biological Dentistry & Medicine
www.IABDM.org

Holistic Dental Association
www.HolisticDental.org

Find a Mercury Free Dentist, Mercury News, Consumer Information, Share Your Story, Mercury Toxicity Questionnaire, Holistic Health Topics

www.TALKInternational.com

Consumer Organizations

DAMS – Dental Amalgam Mercury Solutions www.amalgam.org

Consumers for Dental Choice www.ToxicTeeth.org

Californians for Green Dentistry
www.facebook.com/californiansforgreendentistry

Mercury Free Baby www.MercuryFreeBaby.org

The Pregnant Dentist   www.PregnantDentist.org

CoMeD - The Coalition for Mercury-free Drugs
www.mercury-freedrugs.org

Fluoride Action Network www.fluoridealert.org

The Mercury Policy Project www.mercurypolicy.org

Mercury Victims Websites

www.MercuryPoisoned.com

www.poisonmetal.com

Information about Mercury in Dentistry

Collection of studies and regulatory actions related to dental mercury fillings: www.library.iaomt.org

IAOMT Position Paper:
http://iaomt.org/wp-content/uploads/IAOMT-2013-Position-Statement.pdf

www.MercuryExposure.info

Online Biological Dentistry Education – for Dental Professionals and Consumers

www.BiologicalCE.com

Interactive Meridian Tooth Chart

www.MeridianToothChart.com

Bio-Compatibility Testing

Clifford Materials Reactivity Testing www.ccrlab.com

Dental DNA Testing www.hugginsappliedhealing.com

Ceramic Implants

Z-Systems www.zsystems.com/en.html

Detoxification Methods and Professionals

Natural Detoxification through exercise:
www.FreedomSpringSystem.com

Hans Gruenn, MD www.DrGruenn.com (Los Angeles)

Dr. Joseph Sciabbarrasi www.DrJosephMD.com (Los Angeles)

Quick Silver Scientific www.quicksilverscientific.com

Mercury Safe Dental Office Equipment
Amalgam Separators

www.MarsBioMed.com

Air Purification and Vacuum Systems

www.Foustco.com

www.MarsBioMed.com

www.DentAirVac.com

Mercury Vapor Monitoring Equipment

Assay Technologies www.assaytech.com

Jerome Vapor Analyzer www.azic.com

About Dr. Rota

Blog: www.Bouncercise.com

Book website: www.MirrorOfTheBody-Book.com

YouTube Channel: www.youtube.com/user/DrJamesRota

Holistic Health/Integrative Medicine Organizations

American College for Advancement in Medicine www.ACAM.org

American Academy of Environmental Medicine
www.AAEMonline.org

Governmental Agencies

Environmental Protection Agency – EPA   www.epa.gov/mercury

Food & Drug Administration – FDA www.fda.gov

MedWatch: The FDA Safety Information and Adverse Event
Reporting Program: www.accessdata.fda.gov/scripts/medwatch

FDA Consumer Complaint Coordinators:
www.fda.gov/Safety/ReportaProblem/ConsumerComplaintCoordinators

United Nations Environmental Programme – Minamata
Convention on Mercury
www.unep.org/chemicalsandwaste/Metals/Mercury

Occupational Safety & Health Administration – OSHA: File a complaint: www.osha.gov/as/opa/worker/complain.html

American Dental Association

Trade Organization   www.ada.org

Consumers   www.MouthHealthy.org

Foundation www.adafoundation.org

Dental Amalgam Manufacturers & Suppliers

Kerr Dental www.kerrdental.com

Dentsply www.dentsply.com

Goldsmith and Revere, Inc. - distributed through Henry Schein

Ivoclar Vivadent www.ivoclarvivadent.us

SDI, Inc. www.sdi.com.au/en-us

Henry Schein www.HenrySchein.com

Dental Board of California - Materials Fact Sheet

www.dbc.ca.gov/formspubs/pub_dmfs_english_webview.pdf

Seafood Safety Updates

Seafood Watch www.seafoodwatch.org

Fish Watch www.fishwatch.gov

Holistic Health Resources

www.Mercola.com

Weston Price Foundation www.westonaprice.org

Money in Politics Information

Center for Responsive Politics www.opensecrets.org

Recommended Reading

(Visit www.TALKInternational.com/media-library/recommended-reading for updated reading lists)

The Toxic Time Bomb - by Sam Ziff

It's All in Your Head: Diseases Caused by Silver-Mercury Fillings - by Dr. Hal Huggins

Uniformed Consent – by Dr. Hal Huggins & Dr. Thomas Levy

The Natural Mind – by Dr. Andrew Weil

Let the Tooth be Known – by Dr. Dawn Ewing

Healing is Voltage: The Handbook – by Dr. Jerry Tennant

Root Canal Cover Up – by Dr. George Meinig

Whole Body Dentistry – by Dr. Mark Breiner

The Poison in Your Teeth – by Dr. Tom McGuire

Cure for All Diseases – by Dr. Hulda Clark

Alternative Medicine, the Definitive Guide

Tooth Truth – by Dr. Frank Jerome

The Terrain is Everything – by Susan Stockton

Surviving the Toxic Crisis – by Dr. William Kellas and Dr. Andrea Dworkin

Recommended Videos

"Evidence of Harm" – www.evidence-of-harm.com

Panorama – "Poisons in Your Mouth"

60 Minutes, "Is There Poison in Your Mouth?"

www.talkinternational.com/media-library/video-library

"Mercury Undercover" – www.mercuryundercover.com

"Fluoridegate" - www.fluoridegate.com

"Trace Amounts" – www.traceamounts.com

Referenced Literature

(in order of referral)

Stock A. [Zeitschrift fuer angewandte Chemie, 29. Jahrgang, 15. April 1926, Nr. 15, S. 461-466, Die Gefaehrlichkeit des Quecksilberdampfes, von Alfred Stock (1926).] The Dangerousness of Mercury Vapor. Translated by Birgit Calhoun. http://www.stanford.edu/~bcalhoun/AStock.htm.

Kilpatrick, Harold C. Work Simplification in Dental Practice: Applied Time and Motion Studies 25 Contributing Authors. Philadelphia: Saunders, 1964. Print.

Ziff, Sam. The Toxic Time Bomb: Mercury Amalgam Dental Fillings. Wellingborough: Thorsons, 1985. Print.

Huggins, Hal A. It's All in Your Head: Diseases Caused by Silver-mercury Fillings. 4th ed. Place of Publication Not Identified: Life Sciences, 1990. Print.

Weil, Andrew. The Natural Mind: A New Way of Looking at Drugs and the Higher Consciousness. Boston: Houghton Mifflin, 1972. Print.

Mutter J. Is dental amalgam safe for humans? The opinion of the scientific committee of the European Commission. Journal of Occupational Medicine and Toxicology. 2011; 6:2.

Eggleston DW, Nylander M.; Correlation of dental amalgam with mercury in the brain. J Prost Dent 1987;58:704-707

Retrograde Axonal Transport of Mercury; Bjoern Arvidson Experimental Neurology 1987;98, 198-203

Inorganic Mercury is Transported from Muscular Nerve Terminals to Spinal and Brainstem Motorneurons: Bjoern Arvidson Muscle and Nerve 1992;15:1089-1094

S.Hussain et al, "Mercuric chloride-induced reactive oxygen species and its effect on antioxidant enzymes in different regions of rat brain",J Environ Sci Health B 1997 May;32(3):395-409

Stohs SJ, Bagchi D. Oxidative mechanisms in the toxicity of metal ions. Free Radic Biol Med 1995; 18(2): 321-36

Yannai S, Berdicevsky I, Duek L. Transformations of inorganic mercury by candida albicans and saccharomyces cerevisiae. Applied and Environmental Microbiology. 1991; 57(1):245-247.

Zamm AV. Removal of dental mercury: Often an effective treatment for the very sensitive patient. J Orthomol Med. 1990; 5(3):138-142.

Colson DG. A safe protocol for amalgam removal. J Environ Public Health. 2012;2012:517391. Epub 2012 Jan 18.

Gonzalez-Ramirez D, Maiorino RM, Zuniga-Charles M, Xu Z, Hurlbut KM, Junco-Munoz P, Aposhian MM, Dart RC, Diaz Gama JH, Echeverria D. Sodium 2, 3-dimercaptopropane-1-sulfonate challenge test for mercury in humans: II. Urinary mercury, porphyrins and neurobehavioral changes of dental workers in Monterrey, Mexico. Journal of Pharmacology and Experimental Therapeutics. 1995; 272(1):264-274.

Vandenberge, John et al. Blood serum mercury test report. The Journal of the American Dental Association, 1977; Volume 94, Issue 6, 1155 - 1157J Am Dent Assoc. 1977 Jun ;94(6):1155-7.

Ritchie KA, Burke FJ, Gilmour WH, Macdonald EB, Dale IM, Hamilton RM, McGowan DA, Binnie V, Collington D, Hammersley R. Mercury vapour levels in dental practices and body mercury levels of dentists and controls. Br Dent J. 2004;197(10):625-32; discussion 621.

Guyton, Arthur C., and John E. Hall. Textbook of Medical Physiology. 9th ed. Philadelphia: Saunders, 1996. Print.

"Basic Information." EPA. Environmental Protection Agency. Web. 20 June 2015.

"Thread: CRAWCOUR -SURGEON DENTISTS -ENGLAND." British Genealogy Family History Forums RSS. Web. 10 June 2015.

"Dental Quackery : An Address before the American Dental Convention at Niagara Falls, August 5 1859 : Wilson, E.T." Internet Archive. Web. 3 July 2015.

Hyson, JM. "Amalgam: Its History and Perils." CDA Journal 34.3 (2006): 215. Print.

Koch, Charles R. E., and Burton Lee Thorpe. History of Dental Surgery:. Chicago: National Art Pub., 1909. Print.

Transactions of the American Dental Association. Cleveland: Association, 1863. Print.

British Journal of Dental Science and Prosthetics. Vol. 47. London, 1901. Print.

History of Dental Surgery, Volume 2 By Charles Rudolph Edward Koch, Burton

Bethel, MD, DDS, L.P. The Dental Summary. Vol. 42. 1922. Print.

"Chapin A. Harris." Wikipedia. Wikimedia Foundation. Web. 16 June 2015.

The New England Journal of Dentistry and Allied Sciences. Vol. 1. Springfield: New England Journal., 1882. Print.

Mezei, Ernie. "Tooth Traitors." TALK International Article Tooth Traitors Comments. Web. 9 Sept. 2015.
<http://www.talkinternational.com/articles-research/article-tooth-traitors/>.

"Safety Data Sheet acc. To OSHA HCS, Version number 2, Printed 08/11/2014

"Fillings (Silver-Colored)." Silver Colored Fillings. Web. 8 Aug. 2015.
<http://www.mouthhealthy.org/en/az-topics/f/fillings-silver-colored>.

Sellars WA, Sellars R. Univ. Of Texas Southwestern Medical School "Methyl mercury from dental amalgams in the human mouth", Journal of Nutritional & Environmental Medicine 1996
Heintze et al,"Methylation of Mercury from dental amalgam and mercuric chloride by oral Streptococci".,Scan. J. Dent. Res. 1983, 91:150-152

Harris HH, Vogt S, Eastgate H, Legnini DG, Hornberger B, Cai Z, Lai B, Lay PA. Migration of mercury from dental amalgam through human teeth. J Synchrotron Radiat. 2008;15(Pt 2):123-8.

"Methylmercury." Definition Page. Web. 14 July 2015.
<http://toxics.usgs.gov/definitions/methylmercury.html>.

Pleva, PhD, Jero. "Corrosion and Mercury Release from Dental Amalgam." Journal of Orthomolecular Medicine 4.3 (1989). Print.

"Safe Removal of Amalgam Fillings." IAOMT.org. IAOMT. Web. 3 Aug. 2015. <http://iaomt.org/safe-removal-amalgam-fillings/>.

"Minamata Convention on Mercury." United Nations, 1 Oct. 2013. Web. 13 Sept. 2015. <http://www.mercuryconvention.org/Portals/11/documents/Bookle ts/Minamata Convention on Mercury_booklet_English.pdf>.

"Mercury in Dental Amalgam." EPA. Environmental Protection Agency. Web. 17 Aug. 2015. <http://www.epa.gov/mercury/dentalamalgam.html>.

"EPA Proposed Amalgam Separator Rule." EPA Proposed Amalgam Separator Rule | Open4BioClean. Web. 1 Oct. 2015. <http://open4bioclean.com/forum/waste-water-dental/epa-proposed-amalgam-separator-rule>.

"EPA Will Propose Rule to Protect Waterways by Reducing Mercury from Dental Offices/Existing Technology Is Available to Capture Dental Mercury." 09/27/2010: Web. 29 Aug. 2015.

"EU Should Curb Mercury Emissions from Cremations, Campaigners Say." Reuters. Thomson Reuters, 12 Jan. 2015. Web. 17 Aug. 2015.

McCracken MS, Gordan VV, Litaker MS et al. A 24-month evaluation of amalgam and resin-based composite restorations. JADA 2013; 144, 583-593.

Miller, EG, et. al. Prevalence of mercury hypersensitivity in dental students. J Dent Res. 64: Special Issue, p. 338, Abstact #1472, (1985).

White RR, Brandt RL. Development of mercury hypersensitivity among dental students. JADA. 1976; 92(6):1204-7.

Koral S. The Scientific Case against Amalgam. Champion'sGate, FL: IAOMT. 2005.

"Statement on Dental Amalgam." Statement on Dental Amalgam. American Dental Association, 1 Aug. 2009. Web. 10 Aug. 2015.

Brown, Charlie. "Banner Year 2001-02." Consumers for Dental Choice, 2002. Web. 1 Oct. 2015. <http://www.toxicteeth.org/bannerYear01-02.aspx>.

Kaitlin McGrath, A Toxic Mouthful: the Misalignment of Dental Mercury Regulations, 33 B.C.J.L. & Soc. Just. 347 (2013), http://lawdigitalcommons.bc.edu/jlsj/vol33/iss2/4>.

"Veracity." Veracity. American Dental Association. Web. 9 Aug. 2015. <http://www.ada.org/en/about-the-ada/principles-of-ethics-code-of-professional-conduct/veracity>.

"CALIFORNIA'S COMPLIANCE WITH DENTAL AMALGAM DISCLOSURE POLICIES." U.S. Government Printing Office, 26 Jan. 2004. Web. 3 Sept. 2015. <http://www.gpo.gov/fdsys/pkg/CHRG-108hhrg93640/html/CHRG-108hhrg93640.htm>.

"Dental Materials Fact Sheet." Dental Board of California, 2004. Web. 18 Aug. 2015.
<http://www.dbc.ca.gov/formspubs/pub_dmfs2004.pdf>.

Legal brief filed in W.H. Tolhurst vs. Johnson & Johnson Consumer Products, Inc; Engelhard Corp.; ABE Dental Inc.; The American Dental Association, et al. In the Superior Court of the State of California, In and For the Country of Santa Clara. Case No. 718228. 1995.

"Jim Love Introduction, Story of the Tolhurst Case and ADA Owing No Duty of Care to the Public." YouTube, 20 July 2011. Web. 18 Aug. 2015.

"About Dental Amalgam Fillings." U.S. Food and Drug Administration. Web. 19 Aug. 2015.

Cartland, Robert. "The US Dental Amalgam Debate, 2010 Meeting of the FDA Dental Products Panel." IAOMT.org. 2011. Web. 1 Aug. 2015. <http://iaomt.org/wp-content/uploads/Cartland-US-Dental-Amalgam-Debate-2010-FDA-Meeting-2012-11-18.pdf>.

T. Willumsen, "Dental fear in sexually abused women," European Journal of Oral Sciences, vol. 109, no. 5, pp. 291–296, 2001

Th. Leventouri, A. Antonakos, A. Kyriacou, R. Venturelli, E. Liarokapis, and V. Perdikatsis, "Crystal Structure Studies of Human Dental Apatite as a Function of Age," International Journal of Biomaterials, vol. 2009, Article ID 698547, 6 pages, 2009.

Kramer: Energetic Interrelations between Maxillo-Dental Region & Whole Organism. Web. 8 Sept. 2015.
<http://www.biologicaldentalhealth.com/dr-verigins-biodental-library/84.html>.

Voll R. *Verification of acupuncture by means of electroacupuncture by Voll.* Am J Acupuncture 1977;6: 5-15

Tiller, W.A.: *What do electrodermal diagnosis acupuncture instruments really measure?* Amer. J. Acupuncture Vol. 15, No. 1 March 1987, pp 15-23.

Voll R.: *Twenty years of electroacupuncture diagnosis in Germany. A progress report.* Amer. J. Acupuncture 1975;3 (19)

"Interactive Meridian Tooth Chart." TALKInternational Meridian Tooth Chart. American Bio-Compatible Health Systems, Inc. Web. 19 Aug. 2015. <http://www.talkinternational.com/meridian-tooth-chart/>.

Ewing, Dawn. Let the Tooth Be Known. Houston, TX: Holistic Health Alternatives, 1998. Print.

Tennant, Jerry. Healing Is Voltage: The Handbook. 3rd ed. CreateSpace Independent Platform, 2010. Print.

Pigatto PDM, Brambilla L, Ferrucci S, Guzzi G. Systemic allergic contact dermatitis due to galvanic couple between mercury amalgam and titanium implant. Skin Allergy Meeting. 2010.

Mumford JM. Electrolytic action in the mouth and its relationship to pain. J Dent Res. 1957; 36(4):632-40.

Bánóczy J, Roed-Petersen B, Pindborg JJ, Inovay J. Clinical and histologic studies on electrogalvanically induced oral white lesions. Oral Surg Oral Med Oral Pathol. 1979; 48(4): 319-23.

"Potential Risks and Side Effects of Dental Implants." Online Surgery. Web. 3 Sept. 2015. <http://www.onlinesurgery.com/article/potential-risks-and-side-effects-of-dental-implants.html>.

Injury of the Inferior Alveolar Nerve during Implant Placement: a Literature Review, Oral Maxillofac Res 2011 (Jan-Mar) vol. 2, No 1.

Metal-Free Dental Implants: A New Approach to Implantology, The New Zealand Charter Journal, Spring 2004. <http://www.z-systems.co.nz/PDFs/nzcharter.pdf>.

Oliva J, Oliva X, Oliva JD, Int J Oral Maxillofac Implants. "Five-year success rate of 831 consecutively placed Zirconia dental implants in humans: a comparison of three different rough surfaces." 2010 Mar-Apr;25(2):336-44.

Depprich R, Ommerborn M, Zipprich H, Naujoks C, Handschel J, Wiesmann HP, Kübler NR, Meyer U."Behavior of osteoblastic cells cultured on titanium and structured zirconia surfaces." Head Face Med. 2008 Dec 8;4:29.

Manicone PF, Rossi Iommetti P, Raffaelli L, Paolantonio M, Rossi G, Berardi D, Perfetti G., Int J "Biological considerations on the use of zirconia for dental devices", Immunopathol Pharmacol. 2007 Jan-Mar;20(1 Suppl 1):9-12.

Lebedev KA, Poniakina ID. "The center of pathological (toxic) action of metals in people organisms and a role of galvanic currents in its induction." Fiziol Cheloveka. 2011 Jul- Aug;37(4):90-7.

Kucerová H, Dostálová T, Procházková J, Bártová J, Himmlová L. "Influence of galvanic phenomena on the occurrence of algic symptoms in the mouth." Gen Dent. 2002 Jan-Feb;50(1):62-5.

Hisbergues M, Vendeville S, Vendeville P. "Zirconia: Established facts and perspectives for a biomaterial in dental implantology." J Biomed Mater Res B Appl Biomater. 2009 Feb;88(2):519-29.

Chaturvedi TP. "An overview of the corrosion aspect of dental implants (titanium and its alloys)." Indian J Dent Res. 2009 Jan-Mar;20(1):91-8.

Muller KE, Valentine-Thon E. Hypersensitivity to titanium: Clinical and laboratory evidence. Neuro Endocrinol Lett. 2006; 27(Suppl1): 31–35.

"Dr Hal Huggins on Dental Implants and Bone Grafts." The Natural Recovery Plan. Web. 10 Aug. 2015. <http://www.thenaturalrecoveryplan.com/articles/Dr-Hal-Huggins-on-Dental-Implants-and-Bone-Grafts.html>.

Lippert, Lynn, and Lynn Lippert. Clinical Kinesiology and Anatomy. 4th ed. Philadelphia: F.A. Davis, 2006. Print.

Taylor, Joyal. The Complete Guide to Mercury Toxicity from Dental Fillings: How to Find out If Your Silver Dental Fillings Are Poisoning You and What You Can Do about It. San Diego: Scripps, 1988. Print.

"OSHA Standards." Safety and Health Topics | Mercury - OSHA Standards. U.S. Department of Labor - Occupational Safety & Health Administration. Web. 1 Sept. 2015.

Gerhard I, Frick A, Monga B: Diagnosis of mercury body burden. Clin Lab 1997;43:637-647

Windham, Bernard. "The Role of Mercury in Periodontal Disease and Oral Health Problems." The Natural Recovery Plan. Web. 15 Sept. 2015.

"Basic Information." EPA. Environmental Protection Agency. Web. 9 Oct. 2015. <http://www.epa.gov/mercury/about.htm>.

"Safe, Sustainable Seafood." Green America's Real Green Newsletter. Web. 16 Sept. 2015. <http://www.greenamerica.org/livinggreen/seafood.cfm>.

"Consumer and Commercial Products." EPA. Environmental Protection Agency. Web. 23 Aug. 2015. <http://www.epa.gov/mercury/consumer.htm>.

"Exposure to Mercury: A Major Health Concern." Preventing Disease Through Healthy Environments. World Health Organization. Web. 10 Aug. 2015.

Koss, Freya. "Symptoms of Chronic Mercury Poisoning." Mercury Poisoned: Symptoms of Chronic Mercury Toxicity. Web. 14 Sept. 2015. <http://www.mercurypoisoned.com/symptoms.html>.

Clarkson TW, Hursh IB, Sager PR, Sverson TLM: Mercury. In Biological Monitoring of Toxic Metals (Clarkson TW, Friberg L, Nordberg CF,, and Sager PR, eds) pp 199-246. Plenum, New York 1988.

Hultman P, Johansson U, Turley Sj, Lindh U, Enestrom S, Pollard KM; Adverse immunological effects and autoimmunity induced by dental amalgam and alloy in mice. FASEB J 1994;8:1183-1190

Klassen CD. Heavy metals and heavy-metal antagonists. In: The Pharmacological Basis of Therapeutics, 8th edition(Gilman AC, Rall TW, Niew AS, Taylor P, eds) pp. 1598-1602. Pergamon Press, New York 1990.

Nylander M, Frierg I, Lind B; Mercury concentrations in the human brain and kidneys in relation to exposure from dental amalgam fillings. Swed Dent J 1987;11:179-187

Biagazzi M, Pierlguigi E; Autoimmunity and heavy metals. Lupus 1994;3:449-453.

Dondero F, Lenzi A, Lombardo F, Gandini L; Therapy of immunologic infertility. Acta Eur Fertil 1991;22:139-145

Rowlands AS, Baird DD, Weinberg CP, Shore DL, Shy CM, Wilcos AJ. The effect of occupational exposure to mercury vapor on the fertility of female dental assistants. Occup Environ Med 1994;51:28-34.

Gerhard I, Monga B, Waldbrenner A, Runnebaum B Heavy metals and fertility. J Toxicol Environ Health 1998;21;54(8):593-611

Hultman P, Johansson U, Turle S,J, et al: Adverse immunological effects and autoimmunity induced by dental amalgam and alloy in mice. FASEB J 1994;8:1183-1190

Gerhard I, Frick A, Monga B: Diagnosis of mercury body burden. Clin Lab 1997;43:637-647

Siblered TL, Kienholz E. Evidence that mercury from silver dental fillings may be an etiological factor in reduced nerve conduction velocity in multiple sclerosis patients. Journal of Orthomolecular Medicine 1997;12(3):169-172.

Summers AO, Wireman J, Vimy MI, Lorscheider FI, Marshall B, Levy SB, et al; Mercury released from dental silver fillings provokes an increase in mercury and antibiotic-resistant bacteria in oral and intestinal floras of primates. Antimicrob Agents and Chemo 1993;37:825-834

Barregard L, Lindtedt G, Shutz A, et al. Endocrine function in mercury exposed chloralkali workers. Occup Environ Med 1994, 51 (8)536-540.

Moszczynski P, Lisiewica J, Bartus R, et al. Lymphocytes T and NK cells in men occupationally exposed to mercury vapors. Int J Occup Med Environ Health 1995 8(1):49-56.

Siblerud RL; The relationship between mercury from dental amalgam and mental health. Am J Psychotherapy 1989;18:575-587

Escheverria D, Hever N, Martin MD, Naleway CA, Woods JS Bittner AC; Behavioral effects of low level exposure to mercury among dentists. Neurotxicol Teratol 1995;17:161-168

Klinghardt, Richard. "Mercury Toxicity and Systemic Elimination Agents – Information and Sources." Mercola.com. Web. 27 Aug. 2015.

Shade, PhD, Christopher. " What Is Mercury Speciation Analysis?" Mercury Speciation and Detoxification. Web. 11 Aug. 2015. <https://www.quicksilverscientific.com/the-science/what-is-mercury-speciation>.

"Mercury Fillings: What's All the Fuss?" Valley Health Magazine, 3 Feb. 2010. Web. 20 Aug. 2015.

American Dental Association False Claims on Amalgam, Dental Mercury Health Risk." CureZone Educating Instead of Medicating. Web. 21 Aug. 2015. <http://www.curezone.org/dental/dental_claims.asp>.

Ngim CH: Chronic neurobiological effects of elemental mercury in dentists. Br J Indust Med 1992;49:782-790

Mutter J. Is dental amalgam safe for humans? The opinion of the scientific committee of the European Commission. Journal of Occupational Medicine and Toxicology. 2011; 6:2.

Mutter J, Curth A, Naumann J, Deth R, Walach H. Does inorganic mercury play a role in Alzheimer's disease? A systematic review and an integrated molecular mechanism. J Alzheimers Dis. 2010; 22(2):357-74. Review.

Lorscheider FL, Vimy MJ. Evaluation of the saftey issue of mercury release from dental fillings. FASEB J 1993;7:432-1433

Aposhian HV, Aposhia MM. Meso-2,3 dimercaptosuccinic acid: chemical, pharmacological and toxicological properties of an orally effective metal chelating agent. Annu Rev Toxicol 1990;30:279-306

Aaseth J, Jacobsen D, Andersen O, Wickstrom E. Treatment of mercury and lead poisonings with dimercaptosuccinic acid and sodium dimercaptopropanesulfonate. 1995;120(3):853-854

Aposhian HV, Maiorino RM, Rivera M, et al Human studies with the chelating agents, DMPS and DMSA. J Toxicol Clin Toxicol 1992;30(4):505-528

Margaret E. Sears, "Chelation: Harnessing and Enhancing Heavy Metal Detoxification—A Review," The Scientific World Journal, vol. 2013, Article ID 219840, 13 pages, 2013.

Goodrich JM, Wang Y, Gillespie B, Werner R, Franzblau A, Basu N. Glutathione enzyme and selenoprotein polymorphisms associate with mercury biomarker levels in Michigan dental professionals. Toxicology and Applied Pharmacology. 2011; 257(2): 301-308.

Cabaña-Muñoz ME, Parmigiani-Izquierdo JM, Bravo-González LA, Kyung HM, Merino JJ. Increased Zn/Glutathione Levels and Higher Superoxide Dismutase-1 Activity as Biomarkers of Oxidative Stress in Women with Long-Term Dental Amalgam Fillings: Correlation between Mercury/Aluminium Levels (in Hair) and Antioxidant Systems in Plasma. PLoS ONE. 2015;10(6):e0126339.

Fidelus R.K., Tsan M.F. Glutathione and lymphocyte activation: a function of aging and auto-immune disease. Immunology. 1987 61:503-508.

"Disruptions in Natural Body-wide Detoxification." Mercury Research. Quicksilver Scientific. Web. 11 Oct. 2015. <https://www.quicksilverscientific.com/the-science/what-we-discovered>.

Dempster, John. "Top 10 Detoxifying Foods." The Huffington Post. Web. 24 Aug. 2015.

Felts CN, Lauren. "10 Holistic Treatments for Lymphatic System Health." The Chalkboard: Detox Your Lymph 10 Holistic Treatments For Your Lymphatic System Comments. 24 Feb. 2015. Web. 17 Aug. 2015.

Brooks, Kirsten. "The Benefits of Detoxification." The Energy Grid. 1 July 2007. Web. 17 Aug. 2015. <http://www.energygrid.com/health/2007/07kb-detoxification.html>.

Guyton, Arthur C., and John E. Hall. Textbook of Medical Physiology. 10th ed. Philadelphia: Saunders, 2000. Print.

"Dental Filling Materials: Dental Amalgam." American Dental Association. Web. 28 Aug. 2015. <http://www.ada.org/en/member-center/oral-health-topics/amalgam>.

"Statement on Dental Amalgam." American Dental Association. Web. 11 Sept. 2015. <http://www.ada.org/en/about-the-ada/ada-positions-policies-and-statements/statement-on-dental-amalgam>.

"Position Statement against Dental Mercury Amalgam Fillings."
IAOMT.org. IAOMT, 16 Apr. 2013. Web. 16 Aug. 2015.
<http://iaomt.org/wp-content/uploads/IAOMT-2013-Position-Statement.pdf>.

Bellinger DC, Trachtenberg F, Barregard L, et al. Neuropsychological
and renal effects of dental amalgam in children: a randomized clinical
trial. JAMA 2006;295(15):1775-83. Accessed October 9, 2013.

"LITERATURE REVIEW: DENTAL AMALGAM FILLINGS AND HEALTH
EFFECTS, ADA Council on Scientific Affairs." American Dental
Association. Web. 11 Sept. 2015.
<http://www.ada.org/~/media/ADA/Member%20Center/FIles/amal
gam_literature_review_1009.ashx>.

Geier DA, Carmody T, Kern JK, King PG, Geier MR. A dose-dependent
relationship between mercury exposure from dental amalgams and
urinary mercury levels: a further assessment of the Casa Pia
Children's Dental Amalgam Trial. Hum Exp Toxicol. 2012
Jan;31(1):11-7. Epub 2011 Jul 29.

Haley, Boyd. "Response to the NIDCR Funded Children's Amalgam
Testing Publications in the JAMA 2006." Web. 4 Aug. 2015.
<http://iaomt.guiadmin.com/wp-content/uploads/CAT_Haley_scientific_critique.pdf>.

Geier DA, Kern JK, Geier MR. The biological basis of autism
spectrum disorders: Understanding causation and treatment by
clinical geneticists. Acta Neurobiol Exp (Wars). 2010;70(2):209-26.

Al-Saleh I, Al-Sedairi AA. Mercury (Hg) burden in children: the impact
of dental amalgam. Sci Total Environ. 2011 Jul 15;409(16):3003-15.
Epub 2011 May 20.

FDI Policy Statement/WHO Consensus Statement on Dental
Amalgam. September 1997.

ADA Council on Scientific Affairs. Dental Amalgam: Update on Safety
Concerns. J Am Dent Assoc. 1998;129:494-503.

Koral, Stephen. "The Scientific Case Against Amalgam." IAOMT.org.
2005. Web. 10 Aug. 2015.
<http://library.iaomt.org/sites/default/files/document/Koral The
scientific 2005.pdf>.

Saxe SR, Wekstein MW, Kryscio RJ, et al. Alzheimer's disease, dental
amalgam and mercury. J Am Dent Assoc. 1999;130(2):191-9.

Clarkson TW, Magos L, Myers GJ. The toxicology of mercury –
Current exposures and clinical manifestations. N Engl J Med.
2003;349:1731-7.

Brownawell AM, Berent S, Brent RL, et al. The potential adverse
health effects of dental amalgam. Toxicol Rev 2005;24(1):1-10.

Bellinger DC, Trachtenberg F, Barregard L, et al. Neuropsychological
and renal effects of dental amalgam in children: a randomized clinical
trial. JAMA 2006;295(15):1775-83.

Bellinger DC, Daniel D, Trachtenberg F, Tavares M, McKinlay S.
Dental amalgam restorations and children's neuropsychological
function: the New England Children's Amalgam Trial. Environ Health
Perspect 2007;115(3):443-6.

DeRouen TA, Martin MD, Leroux BG, et al. Neurobehavioral effects of
dental amalgam in children: a randomized clinical trial. JAMA
2006;295(15):1784-92.

European Commission: Scientific Committee on Emerging and Newly
Identified Health Risks. The Safety of Dental Amalgam and
Alternative Dental Restoration Materials for Patients and Users May
6, 2008.

Geier DA, Kern JK, Geier MR. A prospective study of prenatal
mercury exposure from maternal dental amalgams and autism
severity. Acta Neurobiol Exp (Wars). 2009;69(2):189-97.

Geier DA, Kern JK, Geier MR. The biological basis of autism
spectrum disorders: Understanding causation and treatment by
clinical geneticists. Acta Neurobiol Exp (Wars). 2010;70(2):209-26.

Hahn, LJ; Kloiber, R; Leininger, RW; Vimy, MJ; Lorscheider, FL.
Dental "silver " tooth fillings: a source of mercury exposure revealed
by whole body scan and tissue analysis. FASEB J, 3:2641-6, 1989.

Hahn, LJ; et al. Whole-Body Imaging of the Distribution of Mercury
Released from Dental Fillings into Monkey Tissues. FASEB J. 4:3256-
609 1990.

Danscher, G; et al. Traces of Mercury in Organs from Primates with
Amalgam Fillings Experim Molec Pathol, 52:291-9, 1990.
Clarkson TW, Friberg L, Hursh JB, Nylander M. The prediction of
intake of mercury vapor from amalgams. In: Clarkson TW, Friberg L,

Nordberg GF, Sager PR, editors. Biological Monitoring of Toxic Metals. New York: Plenum Press; 1988. pp. 247–264.

Ehmann WD, Markesbery WR, Alauddin M, Hossain TI, Brubaker EH. Brain trace elements in Alzheimer's disease. Neurotoxicology Spring; 7(1):195-206 (1986)

Thompson CM, Markesbery WR, Ehmann WD, Mao YX, Vance DE. Regional brain trace-element studies in Alzheimer's disease. Neurotoxicology Spring; 9(1):1-7 (1988)

Wenstrup D, Ehmann WD, Markesbery WR. Trace element imbalances in isolated subcellular fractions of Alzheimer's disease brains. Brain Res Nov 12;533(1):125-31 (1990)

Cornett CR, Markesbery WR, Ehmann WD Imbalances of trace elements related to oxidative damage in Alzheimer's disease brain. Neurotoxicology Jun; 19(3):339-45 (1998)

Basun H, Forssell LG, Wetterberg L, Winblad B. Metals and trace elements in plasma and cerebrospinal fluid in normal aging and Alzheimer's disease. J Neural Transm, Park Dis Dement Sect. 3(4):23

Hock C, Drasch G, Golombowski S, Muller-Spahn F, Willershausen-Zonnchen B, Schwarz P, Hock U, Growdon JH, Nitsch RM.. Increased Blood Mercury Levels in Patients With Alzheimer's Disease. J Neural Transm., 105(1):59-68, (1998).

Leong, C., Syed, N.I. and Lorscheider, F.L. Retrograde degeneration of neurite membrane structural integrity of nerve growth cones following in vitro exposure to mercury. NeuroReport 12(4):733-737, 2001

Pendergrass JC, Haley BE. Inhibition of brain tubulin-guanosine 5'-triphosphate interactions by mercury: similarity to observations in Alzheimer's diseased brain. Met Ions Biol Syst. 1997;34:461-78.

Pendergrass JC, Haley BE, Vimy MJ, et al. Mercury vapor inhalation inhibits binding of GTP to tubulin in rat brain: similarity to a molecular lesion in Alzheimer diseased brain. Neurotoxicology. 1997;18(2):315-24.

Haley BE. The relationship of the toxic effects of mercury to exacerbation of the medical condition classified as Alzheimer's disease. Medical Veritas. 2007; 4(2):1510–1524.

Drasch G, Aigner S, Roider G, Staiger F, Lipowsky G. Mercury in human colostrum and early breast milk. Its dependence on dental amalgam and other factors. J Trace Elem Med Biol. 1998; 12(1):23-7.

Norouzi E, Bahramifar N, Ghasempouri SM. Effect of teeth amalgam on mercury levels in the colostrums human milk in Lenjan. Environ Monit Assess. 2012; 184(1):375-380.

Laks DR. Assessment of chronic mercury exposure within the US population, National Health and Nutrition Examination Survey, 1999–2006. Biometals. 2009; 22(6): 1103-1114.

Richardson GM, Wilson R, Allard D, Purtill C, Douma S, Gravière J. Mercury exposure and risks from dental amalgam in the US population, post-2000. Sci Total Environ. 2011 Sep 15;409(20):4257-68.

Hanson, Mats. Mercury Bibliography. 4th ed. Orlando, FL: Bio-Probe, 1994. Print.

"American Dental Assn." Opensecrets.org. Center for Responsive Politics. Web. 10 Sept. 2015. <https://www.opensecrets.org/lobby/clientsum.php?id=D000000105&year=2015>.

Capp, Michael. "NYU Goes "amalgam Free"." Mouthing Off. 20 July 2012. Web. 15 Aug. 2015. <http://www.asdablog.com/nyu-goes-amalgam-free/>.

"Mercury and Dental Amalgam." The FASEB Journal, 1 Oct. 1994. Web. 25 Aug. 2015. <http://www.fasebj.org/content/8/13/989.full.pdf>.

"Silver" Fillings Have Mercury and Harm Children. Dir. Mark Geier. IAOMT. Film. <https://youtu.be/hLyqlJwc_eE>.

Index

A

abutment, 85, 88
acidophilus, 39
acupuncture, 27, 34, 79-80
ADA position, 61
adverse event report, 135
AIDS epidemic, 21, 38
allergic, 22, 59-60, 71
allergies, 14, 60, 85, 99
allopathic, 29, 33, 37, 39, 73, 79, 103, 140
alternative therapies, 27
Alzheimer's Association, 125-126
Alzheimer's Disease, 118-120, 124-126
amalgam separator, 54-55, 134
amalgam waste, 54, 96
amalgamator, 29, 50
ambient music, 90
American Dental Association (ADA), 42, 49-50, 52, 55-56, 59-64, 67-70, 72, 75, 83, 113-114, 116-120, 122-123, 125-126, 127, 130, 134-136
American Dental Convention, 49
American Society of Dental Surgeons, (ASDS) 48-49
anxiety, 88, 90-91, 97
Aposhian, Dr., 41
Aristotle, 47
aroma therapy, 27
Assistant Clinical Professor, 21-22
Attention Deficit Disorder, 15
Austria, 123
autism, 116, 125
Autism Society of America, 125
autoimmune diseases, disorders, 84-86, 99

B

basement, 13
biofeedback, 27, 32
biological dentistry, 32, 34, 77, 83, 128-129, 146
birth defects, 64-66, 68
blockage of energy, 34

blood analysis, 31
blood test, 42
blood-brain barrier, 42
body burden, 41, 87, 104
bonding agents, 57
bone grafts, 86
Bonferroni Correction, 120
Bouncercise, 44-45, 110, 140
BPA, 56
Brazil, 31, 69, 134
brochure, 65-66, 68-69
broken teeth, 57
Brown, Charlie, 62-63
burnout, 37

C

C.N. Johnson Award, 17
California Dental Association (CDA), 63, 65, 67, 68, 74
California Dental Board 62, 64
Californians for Green Dentistry, 63
Canada, 123, 128
cancer, 32, 56, 84, 87, 99, 106, 110-111, 117, 140-141
candida, 39, 99
capsules, 50-51
Cardiovascular Effects, 99
cavitations, 86
Central Nervous System Conditions, 98
ceramic implants, 86
chelating agents, 42
chelation, 105
chewing gum, 94, 114
children, 13, 16-17, 55, 73, 114-117, 122-124
chlorella, 43, 107-108
Chronic Fatigue Syndrome, 37, 85
chronic mercury exposure, 117, 125, 141
chronic mercury poisoning, 94, 103
cilantro, 43, 107-108
circulation, 34, 43, 82, 111, 139, 141-142
city councils, 63
Civil War, 49
Clarkson, Thomas W., 119
Class I, 71
Class II, 71-72
Class III, 71-72
code of ethics, 62

Cognitron, 25-26
colon, 39-40, 87, 106-107
colonics, 39, 106-107, 140-141
composite filling, 54, 57, 124
consumer groups, 55, 71
Consumers for Dental Choice,
50, 55, 62
Costa Mesa, 63
cranial nerves, 78
Crawcour, 48-49
cremation, crematoriums, 55, 96
crystals, 78
Cuban Missile Crisis, 20

D

DAMS, 50, 134
Dawson, Paul, 21
deceptive, 48
delivery system, 19, 26
Denmark, 121, 123, 126
dental assistant, 39, 51, 53, 90-92,
148
dental burs, 147
dental manufacturers, 23, 61
Dental Materials Fact Sheet, 64-65
dental morphology, 22
Dental Products Panel, 71, 124
dental schools, 70, 129-130
dentin, 78, 83
dentinal tubules, 83
depression, 37-38, 84-85, 98, 103
detoxification, 42-44, 83, 100-101,
103-111, 140-141, 144
digestive issues, 84, 93
dimethyl mercury, 47
dissimilar metals, 80-81, 139
DMPS, 41-43, 101, 103, 105, 107,
109
DMSA, 43, 101, 105
DNA analysis, 86
documentary, 130-131, 136
duty of care, 67-70

E

electrical currents, 35, 81-82, 85
electro-acupuncture, 27, 79
electromagnetic, 34, 79-80
elemental mercury, 50, 81, 93

Endocrine and Reproductive Effects,
100
enemas, 106-107
England, 48, 118
Environmental Precautions, 51
EPA, 54-55, 66, 95
epidemic, 21, 38, 59
Epsom salts, 107
Epstein-Barr Syndrome, 37
ergonomic, 22-23, 25-26
estrogen, 117
ethyl-mercury, 93
Evidence of Harm, 131, 136
excrete, 60
excreter, 93
exercise system, 44

F

FDA, 67-72, 114, 124-126, 134-135
fetal, 122
fibromyalgia, 98, 103, 140
Finland, 123
First Amalgam War, 49
fish, 43, 55, 71, 95-96, 104, 107, 116
flora, 39
fluoride, 75, 85, 128
foods, 19, 40, 42-43, 103, 106-108
four-handed dentistry, 23
France, 123
Freedom Spring, 44, 141

G

gag rule, 62
galvanic reaction, 80, 87
galvanism, 80-81, 83, 85
garlic, 43, 106-107, 109
Gastrointestinal Effects, 99
genetic predisposition, 60, 93, 100
Germany, 49, 79, 123
Glutathione, 105-106
gold crown, 80, 82
gold filling, 56
gold watch, 14, 81
grandfathered, 67, 70, 114
Great Lakes Naval Training Center,
17
Greene, Eileen, 26
Gruenn, Hans, 41, 127
Gulf War, 54, 130

H

Haley, Boyd, 116, 119, 125
Hamburg, Martha, 72
handpieces, 23, 26, 147
Hanson, Mats, 125
Hazardous Materials team, 14
Head, Neck and Oral Cavity
Disorders, 98
health history, 82, 104
heavy metal toxicity, 41, 97, 100-101, 103, 128
hemorrhage, 18
Henry Schein, 51, 72
herpes simplex, 29
HMIS Rating, 51
Hoku Point, 89
Holistic Dental Association (HDA), 32, 50
holistic dentistry, 34
holistic physicians, 100
homeopathic, 49, 91
Huggins, Hal 31-32, 59, 63, 86-87, 110, 128
Hunt, Valerie 32
hydrogen sulfide, 81
hydrotherapy, 106
hypnotherapy, 27

I

IAOMT position paper, 134
Immunological Symptoms, 99
implant crown, 88
inert, 21, 47, 59
inflammation, 49, 79, 81, 85
injection, 14, 89-91
inorganic mercury, 93-94, 101
insomnia, 44, 98
insurance companies, 33, 53-54, 135
International Academy of Biological
Dentistry & Medicine (IABDM), 32, 50, 129, 135
International Academy of Oral
Medicine & Toxicology (IAOMT), 32-33, 41, 50, 53, 55, 113-114, 120, 122-124, 129, 134-135
iridology, 27
It's All in Your Head, 32

J

jogging, 37
Johns Hopkins Hospital, 32
Joliet, 15
Joy, Brugh, 32, 139

K

Kemler, 51
Kennedy, David, 122
kidney disease, 99, 116
Kilpatrick, 19-20
kinesiology, 88-89
Kotagal, Suresh, 124
Kramer, Fritz, 79

L

Laks, Dan, 125
Lena, 90
lesion, 29, 124
Leukemia, 30
lifespan, 95
liquid silver, 47
Lisbon, 116
lobbying budget, 127
lobbyists, 62
loupe, 26
Love, Jim, 70
low-income families, 54
Loyola University, 16-17
lungs, 94-95, 114
lymph, 43, 108, 110-111
lymph flow, 43
lymphatic massage, 111
lymphatic system, 43, 83, 110-111, 140

M

Mad Hatter's Disease, 133
Malibu, 63, 146
manufacturer warnings, 51
massage therapy, 27
Material Safety Data Sheet, 51, 54
maternal, 117, 122
Mayo Clinic, 32, 124
memory, 15, 18, 37, 73, 78, 89, 93, 98, 101-102, 118, 128

XYZ

21896850R00105

Printed in Great Britain
by Amazon